*Recent Advances in*

# Obstetrics and Gynaecology

# Recent Advances in Obstetrics and Gynaecology 20
*Edited by John Bonnar*

ISBN 0-443-06022 3

ISSN 0143 6848

NUMBER
**21**

*Recent Advances in*

# Obstetrics and Gynaecology

*Edited by*

## John Bonnar MA MD (Hons) FRCOG FRCP(I)

Emeritus Professor of Obstetrics and Gynaecology, Trinity College,
University of Dublin; Fellow of Trinity College, Dublin;
Trinity Centre for Health Sciences, St James' Hospital Dublin, Ireland

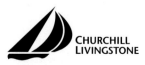

CHURCHILL
LIVINGSTONE

EDINBURGH  LONDON  NEW YORK  PHILADELPHIA  ST LOUIS  SYDNEY  TORONTO  2001

CHURCHILL LIVINGSTONE
An imprint of Harcourt Publishers Limited

First published 2001

ISBN 0-443-06428 8

ISSN 0143 6848

**British Library Cataloguing in Publication Data**
A catalogue record for this book is available from the British Library

**Library of Congress Cataloging in Publication Data**
A catalog record for this book is available from the Library of Congress

Medical knowledge is constantly changing. As new information becomes available, changes in treatment, procedures, equipment and the use of drugs become necessary. The editors and the publishers have, as far as possible, taken care to ensure that the information given in this text is accurate and up to date. However, readers are strongly advised to confirm that the information, especially with regard to drug usage, complies with current legislation and standards of practice.

Commissioning Editor – Ellen Green
Project Editor – Michele Staunton
Project Controller – Frances Affleck
Designer – Sarah Cape
Typeset by BA & GM Haddock

The
publisher's
policy is to use
paper manufactured
from sustainable forests

Printed in Spain

# Contents

# Preface

This 21st issue of *Recent Advances in Obstetrics and Gynaecology* marks the 70th anniversary of the publication. The book is for the specialist registrar and consultant to keep abreast of main developments in obstetrics and gynaecological practice. All of the authors are recognised as experts in their particular field and they provide a concise distillation of their particular topic including 'key points' for clinical practice.

The obstetric section begins with John Spencer of Northwick Park Hospital, London, who has devoted great effort into improving the understanding and interpretation of cardiotocography. This is based on many years of experience in teaching the physiological principles which are the basis of CTG interpretation. Epilepsy continues to be a cause of great concern in a pregnant woman with 19 maternal deaths attributed to epilepsy in the most recent Confidential Enquiry into Maternal Deaths. Bridgette Byrne from the Coombe Women's Hospital, Dublin, reviews the current knowledge aimed at improving the safety of the mother and baby. Ronnie Lamont and colleagues, also from Northwick Park Hospital, continue with an analysis of the place of antibiotics in the prevention of preterm birth and reduction of neonatal morbidity and mortality. We strive to maintain a high standard of clinical management in obstetric emergencies and one of the most important is the management of shoulder dystocia. Thomas Baskett from Halifax, Nova Scotia has a long-standing interest in this complication. He provides an excellent historical review with detailed recommendations for prediction and management of shoulder dystocia. Another emergency, which is a particular hazard in developing countries, is postpartum haemorrhage. Justus Hofmeyr from the University of the Witwatersrand, South Africa, and Metin Gulmezoglu from the World Health Organization in Geneva examine the evidence which has established the effectiveness of active management of the third stage of labour in preventing postpartum haemorrhage, the various pharmacological options and the strategies used to manage postpartum haemorrhage. This is an excellent update which has important implications for both the industrialised and non-industrialised countries.

Shirley Anne Steel from the Peterborough Hospitals Trust has introduced a highly successful risk management programme in the maternity service. This is designed to ensure the highest possible quality of care, with patients being treated in a safe environment and subjected to the minimum risk. I found her definition of quality particularly apt for obstetrics, namely, doing the right thing at the right time and the first time. Her down-to-earth approach is a good example of how risk management can be incorporated into obstetrical practice. Litigation and awards for cerebral palsy account for 40% of the total cost of medical litigation in the National Health Service of England and Wales. Alistair MacLennan of the University of Adelaide has developed an objective template of evidence to allow better identification of cases of cerebral palsy where the neuropathology began or became established around labour and birth. In Australia and New Zealand, he spear-headed a task force aimed at reaching a consensus from scientists, pathologists, neonatologists, midwives, epidemiologists and obstetricians on the causation of cerebral palsy. This was extended to an International Cerebral Palsy Task Force and the Consensus Statement was published in the *British Medical Journal* on 16 October 1999. The Editor of the *British Medical Journal* and Alistair MacLennan kindly agreed to its publication in *Recent Advances in Obstetrics and Gynaecology*. This multi-disciplinary review into the causation and prevention of cerebral palsy is important to every obstetrician and will be of special interest to those who offer expert opinion.

The gynaecology section starts with Andrew Prentice of Cambridge University who contributes an evidence-based analysis of both the medical and surgical treatment of endometriosis-related infertility. Adam Balen from Leeds has a special interest in the laparoscopic treatment of polycystic ovarian syndrome; he offers a detailed review of the literature and the implications for women who have not responded to treatment with Clomiphene. Richard Kennedy, Coventry, presents a detailed analysis of the causes, prevention and treatment of ovarian hyperstimulation syndrome which can be life threatening. He give clear clinical guidance and his algorithm for prevention and management of ovarian hyperstimulation syndrome is recommended as a basis for local protocols in gynaecology units. In recent years, major advances have occurred in the management of male factor infertility. Khaldoun Sharif of Birmingham Women's Hospital, provides a clinically-orientated analysis of male infertility, the clinical assessment of azoospermia and the laboratory investigation and management. This up-date should transform the practice of many gynaecologists who manage the majority of infertile couples outside the specialty of reproductive medicine. More and more women seek the help of gynaecologists for advice on the management of the health issues related to the menopause. Edward Morris and Janice Rymer of Guy's Hospital, London, offer an evidence-based review on the risk benefit ratio of hormone replacement therapy. This chapter will ensure that women are provided with the most up-to-date information on the choice of treatment and minimising unwanted effects.

The final chapter is by Maria van der Burg of the University Hospital, Rotterdam, on interval debulking surgery in advanced ovarian cancer. This had been the subject of a large European study by the Gynaecological Cancer Co-operative Group of the European Organisation. The surgical complications were minimal and no mortality or severe morbidity due to interval debulking surgery was observed. The large randomised trial showed that interval debulking surgery significantly increased the progression free and overall survival. These large European trials, similar to the trials in North America, are an important way in which every gynaecological oncologist can participate and, thereby, advance knowledge in the treatment of ovarian cancer.

I would like to express my gratitude to Dr Gill Haddock, Managing Editor and all the contributors to the 21st issue of *Recent Advances in Obstetrics and Gynaecology* and the first issue of the new millennium. The first Editor of this series was Alec Bourne and in his Preface published in 1930, he wrote: 'while it is necessary to describe new work, it perhaps is even more important to record movements of thought and trends of opinion'. I am sure that this issue of *Recent Advances in Obstetrics and Gynaecology* will keep you, the readers, abreast of the main developments in obstetric and gynaecological practice in both industrialised and non-industrialised countries and so assist you to provide the best and most up-to-date treatment for your patients.

**Dublin 2000**                                                                                 **J. B.**

# Contributors

**Paul E. Adinkra** MBBS
Clinical Research Fellow, Department of Obstetrics and Gynaecology, Northwick Park Hospital and St Mark's NHS Trust, Harrow, Middlesex, UK

**Adam Balen** MB BS MD MRCOG
Consultant in Reproductive Medicine and Honorary Senior Lecturer, Department of Obstetrics and Gynaecology, The General Infirmary, Leeds, UK

**Thomas F. Baskett** MB FRCS(C) FRCS(Ed) FRCOG
Professor, Department of Obstetrics and Gynaecology, Dalhousie University, Halifax, Nova Scotia, Canada

**John Bonnar** MA MD(Hons) FRCP(I) FRCOG
Emeritus Professor of Obstetrics and Gynaecology, Trinity College, University of Dublin, Ireland; Fellow of Trinity College, Dublin; Trinity Centre for Health Sciences, St James' Hospital, Dublin, Ireland

**Bridgette Byrne** MD MRCP(I) MRCOG
Lecturer in Obstetrics and Gynaecology, University College Dublin, Coombe Women's Hospital, Dublin 8, Ireland

**A. Metin Gülmezoglu** MD PhD
UNDP/UNFPA/WHO/World Bank Special Programme of Research, Development and Research Training in Human Reproduction, Department of Reproductive Health and Research, World Health Organization, Geneva, Switzerland

**G. Justus Hofmeyr** MB BCH MRCOG
Professor of Obstetrics and Gynaecology and Director, Effective Care Research Unit, University of the Witwatersrand, South Africa; Obstetrician/Gynaecologist, Cecila Makiwane Hospital and Frere Maternity Hospital, East London, South Africa

**Richard Kennedy** FRCOG
Consultant Obstetrician and Gynaecologist; Honorary Senior Lecturer, Centre for Reproductive Medicine, Walsgrave Hospitals NHS Trust, Coventry, UK

**Ronnie F. Lamont** BSc MD FRCOG
Visiting Reader, Imperial College School of Medicine, London, UK and Consultant, Department of Obstetrics and Gynaecology, Northwick Park Hospital and St Mark's NHS Trust, Harrow, Middlesex, UK

**Alastair MacLennan** MBChB MD FRACOG
Professor of Obstetrics and Gynaecology, University of Adelaide, Women's & Children's Hospital, North Adelaide, South Australia, Australia

**M. Ruth Mason** BSc MBChB
Clinical Research Fellow, Department of Obstetrics and Gynaecology, Northwick Park Hospital and St Mark's NHS Trust, Harrow, Middlesex, UK

**Edward P. Morris** BSc MBBS MRCOG
Specialist Registrar and Honorary Lecturer, Guy's, King's and St Thomas' Medical School, HRT Research Unit, Guy's Hospital, London, UK

**Andrew Prentice** BSc MA MD MRCOG
Consultant Gynaecologist and University Lecturer, Department of Obstetrics and Gynaecology, University of Cambridge, The Rosie Hospital, Cambridge, UK

**Janice Rymer** MBChB MD MRCOG FRNZCOG
Senior Lecturer and Consultant, Department of Obstetrics and Gynaecology, Guy's, King's and St Thomas' Medical School, St Thomas' Hospital, London, UK

**Khaldoun Sharif** MBBCh MRCOG MFFP MD
Consultant Obstetrician and Gynaecologist, Director of Assisted Conception Services, Birmingham Women's Hospital, Birmingham, UK

**John A.D. Spencer** MBBS BSc FRCOG
Consultant Obstetrician and Gynaecologist, Northwick Park Hospital; Honorary Senior Clinical Lecturer, Department of Obstetrics and Gynaecology, University College London, London, UK

**Shirley A. Steel** MB BS FRCOG
Consultant Obstetrician and Gynaecologist, Peterborough Hospitals NHS Trust, Peterborough, UK

**Maria E.L. van der Burg** MD PhD
Department of Medical Oncology, University Hospital Rotterdam Dijkzigt, Rotterdam, The Netherlands

Contributors

*John A.D. Spencer*

# Cardiotocographic assessment of fetal well-being in late pregnancy and labour

Use of the fetal heart rate (FHR) to assess fetal well-being has become standard obstetric practice. The signal can be obtained easily by a number of techniques, and modern technology has resulted in monitors that produce good quality records. However, there remains much criticism of continuous FHR monitoring, particularly during labour, because of the increase in intervention that accompanies its use. This may be due to poor understanding of the physiological basis for FHR changes in different situations, or to an intrinsic inability of the FHR to predict fetal well-being without a significant number of false positives and false negatives. During the last 40 years, a wealth of physiological evidence has been derived from animal experiments and clinical experience.

The cardiotocograph (CTG) is a paper record of the continuous FHR plotted simultaneously with a record of uterine activity. Monitoring fetal well-being in this way assumes that uterine activity during labour is a significant threat to fetal oxygenation and that the fetal response to a significant interference in oxygen delivery is recognisable. Thus, the identification of fetal distress would potentially allow the opportunity to consider appropriate management. However, clinical experience currently perpetuates concern over a number of changes in the FHR, some of which have been shown to be physiological variations of normal.[1] Furthermore, there are clear differences of opinion between expert practitioners when it comes to identification and interpretation of CTG records.[2] Overall, the level of understanding is poor and teaching needs to be improved.

This chapter will present a physiological approach to understanding the FHR which has been taught by the author for more than 10 years. Interpretation is based on known physiological principles rather than learned

**John A.D. Spencer** MBBS BSc FRCOG, Consultant Obstetrician and Gynaecologist, Northwick Park Hospital, Harrow, Middlesex HA1 3AJ, UK

pattern recognition.[3] Knowledge of the physiology helps understand why interpretation of the CTG is not easy and yet can be readily achieved in most cases. It also helps to explain why the few trials of clinical experience based on original FHR classification systems appear to have shown little significant clinical advantage. Modern evidence-based practice questions the wide-spread use of CTG monitoring but a new approach is required before we reject the potential value of this simple signal.

## TECHNOLOGY OF FHR MONITORING

### EXTERNAL (ABDOMINAL) TOCOGRAPHY

A record of uterine activity is obtained by using a strain gauge held onto the front of the abdomen by an elasticised band. As the uterine muscle fibres contract and shorten, the uterus shortens along its longitudinal axis with an increase in width. Furthermore, because it is attached to the pelvic floor, the body of the uterus moves forward within the abdomen to line itself up along the longitudinal axis of the pelvis. Thus, the front of the uterus pushes against the anterior abdominal wall as the myometrial fibres pull it into line with the pelvic inlet. This has the effect of increasing the mother's abdominal girth. Maximal effect is obtained if the transducer is placed just below the uterine fundus.

The tocograph transducer comprises a strain gauge within a supportive housing. The central button or plate moves into the housing as the abdominal wall expands and pushes against it. Inward movement of the central button or plate is transduced into upward movement of a pen on the CTG chart recorder. Thus, as the uterus contracts and the fundus pushes against the anterior abdominal wall, expansion of the anterior abdominal wall can be identified by the tocotransducer. Uterine contractions can be recognised by their characteristic shape on the tocograph as the rising signal accelerates and then slows to a peak before falling in reciprocal fashion. The appearance is like a hill unless interfered with by other movements which can also be seen on the tocograph.

The tocograph transducer on the maternal abdomen is capable of recording many other physical movements both from the fetus and mother. Fetal movements are seen as short, spiky upward deflections of the signal. Maternal breathing is commonly seen as a regular oscillation of the signal and this sometimes increases during contractions and sometimes is lost, according to the position of the transducer on the abdomen. Finally, gross body movements of the mother are evident as sudden deviations of the baseline.

The tocograph signal obtained by an abdominal transducer is merely a qualitative indicator of movements (uterine, fetal, maternal) transduced from the surface of the maternal abdomen. The size of any change seen on the CTG trace does not represent strength of the movement. Uterine contraction frequency can be determined, as can the presence of fetal movements (Fig. 1.1). The maternal position can significantly influence whether or not uterine contractions are recorded well. Experience has shown that uterine contractions do not always record well when the mother is lying in the lateral position. Sitting, standing and lying supine seem to be the best positions for external tocography, but the latter is best avoided because of the risk of aorto-caval compression.

# Cardiotocographic assessment of fetal well-being in late pregnancy and labour

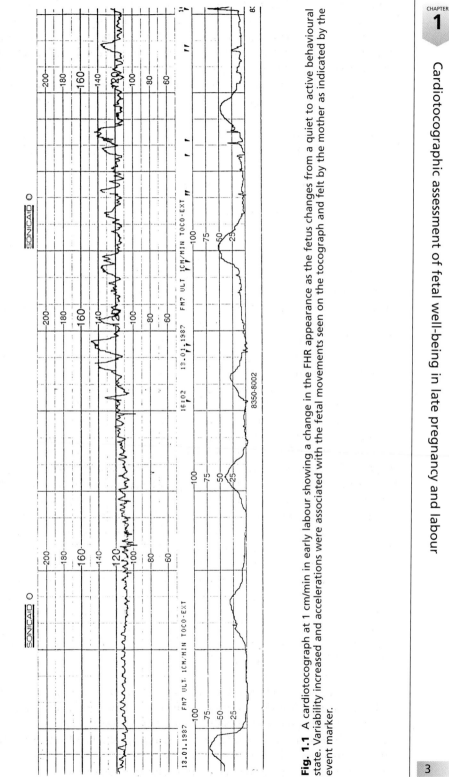

**Fig. 1.1** A cardiotocograph at 1 cm/min in early labour showing a change in the FHR appearance as the fetus changes from a quiet to active behavioural state. Variability increased and accelerations were associated with the fetal movements seen on the tocograph and felt by the mother as indicated by the event marker.

## INTERNAL TOCOGRAPHY

Real measures of uterine contraction pressures can be obtained using an intra-uterine catheter. Early methods involved the use of an intra-uterine fluid-filled cannula to transmit the intra-uterine pressure to a transducer on the monitor. More recently, precalibrated microtransducers attached to the tip of a catheter, suitable for single-use insertion into the uterus, have become available. However, the cost of these is high and the clinical value of intra-uterine pressure measurements remains debatable. Certain clinical situations, such as 'trial of scar', diagnosis of uterine inertia and monitoring the effect of oxytocin augmentation, may benefit from intra-uterine pressure measurements. However, risks of the use of an intra-uterine catheter include trauma and infection which, together with the expense, has resulted in a sharp decline in their routine use during labour.

## EXTERNAL FHR MONITORING

The FHR is most commonly derived from an ultrasound transducer positioned on the maternal abdomen over the fetal heart. Each movement of the beating fetal heart imparts a Doppler shift of the reflected ultrasound, and the resultant waveform is autocorrelated in order to determine the periodicity.[4] This equates with the FHR. By this means any extraneous movements, such as body or breathing movements, are largely prevented from interfering with derivation of the FHR and a clear signal is produced.[5] The main prerequisite is the need to ensure that the ultrasound beam is sited over the heart. A potentially serious complication of this technology is the ability to derive a clean signal from any regular movement. Experience continues to show how easy it can be to obtain a record of the maternal heart rate from the regular pulsations of maternal arteries in the abdomen or pelvis.

Once the transducer is in place, the FHR is usually picked up quite readily. Problems with a good signal can occur if the mother is obese or if the fetus is particularly mobile. Monitoring the premature fetus or when there is polyhydramnios may be particularly difficult. Similarly, if maternal movements become excessive, then there may be significant interruption of the signal. This frequently occurs during the second stage of labour, and local policies should be clear about the need or otherwise for continuous FHR monitoring whilst pushing. If the case is deemed to require this, then consideration may need to be given to monitoring using a fetal scalp electrode.

## INTERNAL FHR MONITORING

The fetal scalp electrode (FSE) is attached directly to the presenting part, and can also be used if the presentation is breech. The electrode is usually in the form of a needle that is designed to penetrate the skin. This ensures that the electrode remains attached whilst also providing good contact with the fetus to pick up the fetal electrocardiogram (ECG). Many attempts have been made to design a commercially viable suction cup plate electrode, but this is not yet commercially available. Use of a FSE has declined since the improvement of ultrasound monitoring following the introduction of autocorrelation. Nevertheless, the need for direct (internal) FHR monitoring will remain an essential backup for cases where external monitoring is unsatisfactory.

The fetal ECG is used to derive the FHR by identification of the R waves. This can sometimes be difficult if the signal is noisy, which may occur when attachment to the skin is loose. The maternal ECG complexes are recognised and removed from the total signal. The resultant fetal signal is usually of good quality and does not depend upon maternal position or activity. However, it is possible to record the maternal heart rate if the fetus is dead. The main disadvantage of this method is the small rate of complications, such as trauma and infection, and the perception that a small needle in the skin of the baby's head is undesirable. To offset these disadvantages the mother does not need a second strap around her abdomen (for the ultrasound transducer) and the quality of the signal is usually better.

Other information can be obtained from the fetal ECG. Several groups are working on aspects of the ECG waveform itself to test the hypothesis that hypoxia may be recognisable before asphyxial damage occurs. Elevation of the ST segment and alterations in the PR/RR interval have been proposed and remain the subject of research. One randomised controlled trial, involving additional information from the ECG waveform in one arm, found a significant reduction in the need for pH sampling in the presence of an abnormal FHR.[6] Whether the negative predictive value will be adequate to allow reliance for monitoring remains to be seen with much larger numbers.

## THE CTG TRACE

The CTG trace is printed at 1 cm/min onto a paper record that is divided into 1 min intervals. Most modern monitors print the time and date at regular intervals, but it is still necessary to ensure appropriate identification of the record with the woman's name and hospital number. It is also useful to check that the wall clock agrees with the time printed on the CTG trace in order to avoid possible confusion at a later date between the CTG and the notes. Once obtained, each trace should be numbered, in order, and reference made to each trace next to the appropriate entry in the notes.

## PHYSIOLOGY OF OXYGEN DELIVERY TO THE FETUS

### UTERO-PLACENTAL PERFUSION

Oxygen reaches the intervillus space via the utero–placental circulation. In early pregnancy, trophoblast invades the decidua and reaches the spiral arteries. Once the vessel has been infiltrated, it is no longer able to offer resistance to flow. The utero–placental vascular bed loses its ability to autoregulate perfusion and blood flow becomes pressure dependent. It is likely that these changes continue well into the second trimester. Utero–placental insufficiency has its origin in the failure of appropriate physiological adaptation of the spiral arteries.[7] The result is that perfusion of the intervillus space remains suboptimal. As a consequence, when increasing fetal requirements surpass the capability of the utero–placental circulation to maintain normal growth, then fetal adaptation begins. This eventually becomes recognised as fetal growth retardation and is characterised by progressive malnutrition and increasing hypoxia leading to asphyxia. However, if the fetus has already reached a good size before placental perfusion becomes inadequate, then fetal growth retardation cannot be recognised. This may explain the difficulty in recognition and under-standing of placental insufficiency at term.

## INTERVILLUS SPACE PERFUSION

Maternal blood flows into the intervillus space from utero–placental arteries. These vessels enlarge as the uterus grows in size, thus facilitating an immense perfusion volume in the absence of resistance to flow. In fact, despite a 30% increase in blood volume, blood pressure still falls in mid-pregnancy. Oxygen delivery to the intervillus space becomes dependent upon utero–placental blood flow, and fetal oxygen and birth weight have been shown to be reduced following reduction of uterine blood flow in various animal models.[8,9] However, uterine perfusion can be reduced quite significantly before fetal hypoxaemia occurs, and fetal acidaemia does not occur until fetal oxygen delivery is reduced below 50%.[10]

The fetus obtains oxygen by diffusion into villus capillaries from maternal blood in the intervillus space. Oxygen delivery may be interrupted acutely by falls in uterine perfusion, such as maternal hypotension or aorto-caval compression. Uterine contractions also reduce utero–placental perfusion,[11] but the significance depends upon background placental function and the frequency of contractions. If there is sufficient time between contractions, then utero–placental perfusion can restore oxygen to the intervillus space even if placental bed vasculature is slightly suboptimal. Nevertheless, in such circumstances, feto-placental reserve is considered reduced, and the fetus may start to develop acidaemia sooner rather than later.

Other acute interruptions of placental perfusion include abruption and uterine hyperstimulation. Both of these conditions may arise on the background of normal placental perfusion. Fetal consequences depend upon the extent to which the delivery of oxygen to the intervillus space is interrupted, and the duration of the interruption. An abruption is a progressive event that may occur slowly or rapidly. Hyperstimulation may be reversed thus allowing restoration of oxygen delivery to the intervillus space.

## UMBILICAL CIRCULATION

Two umbilical arteries bring 50% of the fetal cardiac output to the placenta in a circulation that is parallel to the peripheral circulation in the fetus. Fetal blood leaving the internal iliac arteries passes to capillaries within the placental villi and then leaves the placenta as the non-pulsatile umbilical vein. Oxygen passes from maternal blood in the intervillus space into the umbilical circulation capillaries within the placental villi. Delivery of oxygen from the placenta to the fetus depends upon adequate oxygen in the intervillus space as well as adequate flow in the umbilical vein.[10] Blood returning to the fetus passes through the ductus venosus and joins the vena cava blood entering the right atrium. Thus, blood entering the heart is a mixture of oxygenated blood from the placenta and de-oxygenated blood returning from the fetal periphery. Cord compression is likely to reduce flow in the vein before arterial flow because of the lower pressure within the vessel. Interruptions to venous return will cause a sudden fall in the oxygen level in the blood leaving the fetal heart and reaching the carotid chemoreceptors.

## FETAL RESPONSE TO REDUCED OXYGEN DELIVERY

### FETAL CHEMORECEPTORS

The peripheral arterial chemoreceptors, situated in the neck alongside the carotid artery, are considered to be the sensor of fetal blood oxygen. They receive blood from the heart that is intended for the brain and, therefore, are ideally positioned to respond to changes in arterial oxygen content. Such changes have been modelled in animals[12] and the function of chemoreceptors in the human fetus is presumed to be similar. They are stimulated by changes, rather than a given level, of oxygen in the blood. Thus, it is oxygen delivery that matters rather than the absolute level of fetal arterial oxygen. Interruptions to placental bed perfusion, or cord compression, may result in sufficient reduction in the delivery of oxygen to the fetus that the chemoreceptors are stimulated.

An acute fall in the amount of oxygen in the blood reaching the fetal chemoreceptors (hypoxaemia) results in a transient FHR bradycardia. The carotid sinus nerve conveys the message to the brain stem where stimulation of the vagal nucleus occurs. The vagus nerve is known to convey a chronic slowing influence on the FHR that is balanced by a steady level of sympathetic tone. An acute interruption in oxygen delivery is known to result in a rapid fall in FHR via the vagus nerve, as experiments have shown this to be blocked by atropine and abolished by cutting the vagus. If the reduction in oxygen delivery to the fetus is maintained, but is insufficient to cause acidaemia, then the FHR returns to normal,[13] probably as a result of increasing catecholamine levels from the adrenal glands. This increase in sympathetic stimulation overcomes the effect of the vagal stimulation and also produces a peripheral vasoconstriction. The resulting re-adjustment of the circulation means that the fetal cardiac output becomes more directed towards the brain rather than the peripheral circulation.[14]

### FETAL CATECHOLAMINE SECRETION

If the reduction in oxygen delivery to the fetus is transient, then the changes are readily reversed. Short-lived interruptions in oxygen delivery may not stimulate the adrenal glands and so there may be little rise in catecholamines.

A profound or long-lasting fall in fetal oxygenation produces a significant rise in catecholamine levels.[15] Once oxygen delivery to the fetus is restored, vagal stimulation is reduced and the slowing influence on the FHR is removed. Any circulating catecholamines will then cause an FHR tachycardia that persists until the catecholamine levels return to normal. This may be seen as a 'rebound' tachycardia following a prolonged deceleration.

In the situation of chronic placental insufficiency, fetal arterial oxygenation slowly falls as a result of limited perfusion of the placental bed vessels. The reduction in oxygen delivery to the fetus is slow and does not exceed the rate of fetal adaptation. The slow increase in stimulation of the chemoreceptors is matched by the slow increase in adrenal stimulation. Thus, the increase in both the parasympathetic (slowing) and sympathetic (stimulatory) influences on the FHR occur in parallel and the FHR remains in the normal rate. Variability and accelerations remain normal until the extent of reduction in fetal oxygen delivery becomes severe.[16] Other adaptations include an increase in the haematocrit and reduction in metabolism.[17] Eventually, fetal activity ceases, but FHR accelerations are lost before fetal activity ceases.[18] Shallow FHR decelerations may be seen after uterine tightenings with severe fetal hypoxia, and delivery by Caesarean section becomes imminent.[19]

## FHR MONITORING FOR EVIDENCE OF FETAL HYPOXAEMIA

### FHR MONITORING IN PREGNANCY

#### Indications

Any clinical situation where there is a risk of fetal hypoxaemia is an indication for FHR monitoring. During pregnancy, such situations may be acute or chronic. Acute problems include placental abruption and fetal–maternal haemorrhage. Thus, abdominal pain, antepartum haemorrhage, and a cessation of fetal activity are reasons for performing a CTG. Chronic problems include placental insufficiency, recurrent placental infarction, and rhesus isoimmun-isation. Use of CTG monitoring during pregnancy is usually diagnostic (to obtain information about fetal well-being at that moment) because many studies have shown a lack of clinical efficacy when used for screening or predictive purposes.

Recognition of fetal compromise in the various clinical situations during pregnancy may not be straight-forward. Interpretation of the CTG can only be successful in the context of the reason for performing the test. Thus, acute interruptions of oxygen delivery to the fetus, such as occur with abruption, will be seen as a bradycardia if profound, but, if more slowly progressive, may be seen as reduced variability of a normal baseline, possibly with late decelerations if uterine activity is present.[20] The slower the interruption of oxygen delivery to the fetus, the more likely will be adaptation by the fetus. The ultimate slow hypoxaemia is placental insufficiency. Table 1.1 summarises the mechanisms of interruption to blood flow and the recognisable FHR changes that occur.

Labour is a clinical situation in which the fetus is at greatest risk of having its oxygen delivery interrupted. Not only is uterine activity present (each

**Table 1.1** Common risk factors for fetal hypoxaemia during pregnancy and labour

| Pregnancy | (placental insufficiency) |
| --- | --- |
| | Primiparous |
| | Postmature |
| | Antepartum haemorrhage |
| | Fetal growth retardation |
| | Oligohydramnios |
| | Multiple pregnancy |
| | Maternal vascular disease |
| | Severe hypertension/pre-eclampsia |
| Labour | Uterine hyperstimulation (frequency more than 3 in 10 min) |
| | Prolonged labour |
| | Epidural |
| | Nuchal cord/cord presentation/cord prolapse |

contraction reduces utero–placental perfusion into the intervillus space), but the additional risk of cord compression (reduction of venous return to the fetal heart) exists, especially after rupture of the membranes. It became increasingly common to advocate electronic FHR monitoring routinely during labour, but uncertainty about many of the FHR changes seen has led to a significant association with intervention (operative delivery). Present advice is to use the CTG if the risk for fetal hypoxaemia is significant.[21] The reduction in oxygen delivery to the fetus during labour with unrecognised pre-existing utero–placental insufficiency can be rapid and profound.[22] Rapid changes in FHR are often missed, especially when confined to changes in variability. The idea of screening each fetus in early labour (admission test)[23] to assess the response to uterine activity is based on sound physiological principles and is currently undergoing clinical trials.

### Placental abruption
Abruption can occur at any time during pregnancy or labour. The effect on the FHR depends upon the rate of interference with oxygen delivery. A slow placental separation in labour, with superimposed uterine contractions, will present as late decelerations with diminishing FHR variability. In pregnancy, the loss of variability is likely to precede late decelerations. Once fetal oxygen delivery falls significantly, then FHR becomes bradycardia. This will mean a high chance of severe fetal asphyxia if born alive. Appropriate anticipation in the presence of clinical symptoms and signs results in the best chance of survival provided the abruption has not already progressed too far when first seen.

### Placental infarction
It is possible that a limited area of the placenta becomes damaged, possibly by a small haemorrhage, resulting in an infarct. Many are found after uneventful labour. However, if sufficiently large or recurrent, the possibility that placental function might be reduced must be considered. The acute presentation is characterised by an FHR tachycardia, possibly with reduced variability, that settles over a day or so. Clearly, the differential diagnosis between this and

abruption is merely one of degree and resolution. The FHR must be followed to show that the problem is not progressive. Subsequent management should ensure that fetal growth is maintained.

## Placental insufficiency

This complication of pregnancy probably occurs more often than is clinically recognised. When true fetal growth retardation is diagnosed, then placental insufficiency is highly likely. A small-for-dates fetus is not necessarily growth retarded and may show parallel growth on a lower centile.[24] It is likely that placental insufficiency, however, exists before fetal growth slows down, and animal work suggests that adaptation mechanisms begin before the fetus starts to undergrow. In fact, if placental insufficiency is not severe, then fetal adaptation mechanisms may allow fetal growth to continue. However, fetal reserve will be diminished and tolerance to normal labour may be reduced.

It is believed that the process of fetal adaptation to placental sufficiency is a progressive series of changes, including reduction in fetal activity, reduction in liquor volume and increasing resistance to arterial flow in the umbilical arteries.[25] CTG changes begin with a reduction in accelerations even though fetal movements may still be felt. Decelerations with Braxton-Hicks tightenings occur (see Fig. 1.2), and then variability becomes reduced as oxygenation diminishes further. The FHR remains in the upper normal range. Such FHR decelerations and absent variability is an ominous finding on the CTG,[20,26] occasionally found when a woman presents with a cessation of fetal movements.

## Reduced fetal movements

Reduced fetal activity is a common concern in late pregnancy. However, on some occasions, a cessation of fetal activity is associated with oligohydramnios and CTG evidence of severe placental insufficiency. The risk of intrauterine fetal death is believed to increase after 41 weeks, and this may be evidence of the fact that placental insufficiency may occur in a different manner in late pregnancy. If the fetus has already reached a potentially viable size before placental function is unable to maintain further fetal demands, then fetal adaptation mechanisms at this stage clearly cannot include restriction of growth. Consumption of adipose and glycogen stores may occur, but increasing hypoxaemia may lead to fetal death more abruptly than at earlier gestations. Routine screening of post-date pregnancies has not been shown to be effective. Neither, indeed, has the use of CTG monitoring to investigate fetal movement monitoring.[27]

## 'High risk' pregnancies

The potential for CTG monitoring to recognise fetal adaptation to chronic hypoxia and placental insufficiency has been considered by many to justify prospective screening of pregnancies at increased risk. Unfortunately, the term 'high risk' continues to be abused by its non-specific use with reference to the nature of the risk in question and the likely adverse outcome. FHR monitoring is hardly likely to assist with management of a pregnancy at increased risk of a complication which does not relate to problems with placental function and a reduction in oxygen delivery. Table 1.2 lists common risk factors for fetal hypoxaemia.

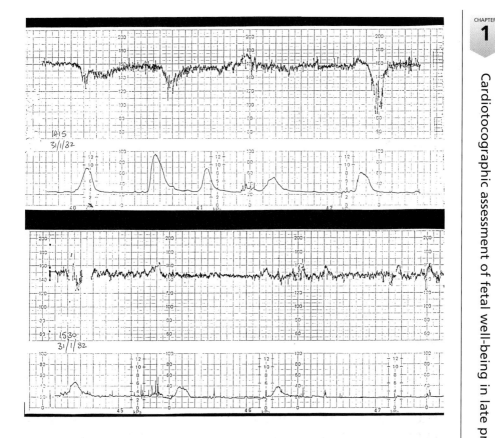

**Fig. 1.2** Two 30 min CTG records at 1 cm/min at 34 weeks, recorded 45 min apart. In the first record, the frequency of (Braxton-Hicks) uterine tightenings produced a slight FHR tachycardia with late decelerations indicating chronic intervillus space hypoxaemia. Note the two FHR accelerations associated with fetal movements (centre of record). The second record shows significant improvement of the FHR as a result of a decrease in frequency of the uterine activity. This illustrates borderline placental insufficiency. Oxygen delivery to the intervillus space, already reduced but still adequate in the absence of uterine activity, became significantly reduced during a run of spontaneous uterine tightenings. A healthy growth-retarded infant was delivered by Caesarean section.

Four randomised controlled trials tested the value of recording the FHR weekly in the antenatal clinic. More of these 'high risk' pregnancies remained out of hospital but there was an almost 3-fold increase in fetal loss if a CTG was performed.[28] Clearly, use of the CTG in this manner may be dangerous. Perhaps the records were too short or the interpretation inexperienced. Perhaps fetal adaptation to chronic hypoxia as a result of placental insufficiency resulted in falsely re-assuring traces. It has been suggested that a CTG needs to be up to 2 h before adequate interpretation is possible. Experience suggests that short out-patient CTG records are only of help if fetal movements are causing concern. Experience with computer-assisted numerical analysis of the CTG is limited, but a number of day assessment units have integrated this in their approach to fetal assessment.

## FETAL MONITORING IN LABOUR

### Indications

From 1980, there was a rapid rise in the use of electronic fetal monitoring.[29] However, in the last 10 years, the limited value of CTG monitoring in all pregnancies has been the subject of much debate. Meta-analysis of the randomised controlled trials suggest some benefit in the form of decreased perinatal loss related to hypoxia, although at the expense of increased operative intervention.[30] From another standpoint, national consensus statements have recommended that the form of monitoring (electronic or auscultation) be selected according to risk status and preference. In the UK, this recommendation was agreed between the RCOG, RCM and RCGP.[21] However, the requirement for good auscultation is one-to-one care during labour and this is rarely achieved in large units. Table 1.2 lists the common causes of fetal hypoxaemia and associated FHR changes.

### Uterine hyperstimulation

Oxygen delivery to the fetus relies upon adequate utero–placental perfusion into the intervillus space.[11] A significant interruption of oxygen delivery to the fetus would produce a deceleration and yet labour proceeds in many women without FHR decelerations. Thus, the reservoir of oxygen in the intervillus space needs to be sufficient to maintain fetal oxygen requirements during intermittent occlusion of utero–placental arteries. Perfusion of the intervillus space resumes between contractions. If uterine contraction frequency is such that perfusion time between contractions does not fully restore intervillus oxygen content, then a progressive hypoxaemia will occur in the intervillus space. Umbilical venous blood will then slowly become hypoxaemic and, eventually, the oxygen content of blood reaching the fetus will fall below a level which triggers a FHR deceleration.

If intervillus space oxygen content falls below the level required to trigger the fetal chemoreceptors, the lowest level will occur at the end, or even shortly after, each contraction. This is because oxygen input (utero–placental perfusion) will have been interrupted during the contraction, but transfer out to the fetal circulation continues. Umbilical blood leaving the placenta becomes progressively hypoxaemic during the contraction and the lowest level of oxygen in the blood reaching the fetal chemoreceptors coincides with the end of each contraction, or even later. Thus, interruptions of oxygen delivery into the intervillus space characteristically produce late FHR decelerations.

### Unrecognised placental insufficiency

It is likely that even normal labour may pose a risk of fetal hypoxaemia in unrecognised placental insufficiency. In such circumstances, intervillus space oxygen content may still be normal in the absence of contractions, or may already be reduced. Perfusion of the intervillus space between contractions will be limited because of the restricted utero–placental flow characteristic of placental insufficiency. Thus, even the unstimulated contractions of normal labour may result in progressive hypoxaemia of the intervillus space with consequent late FHR decelerations. Severe placental insufficiency prior to labour results in sufficient hypoxaemia of the intervillus space to produce late

**Table 1.2** Common causes of fetal hypoxaemia, main effects on the FHR, and clinical management

| Diagnosis | Utero-placental perfusion | Intervillous space oxygen | Umbilical vein blood flow | FHR changes (fetal hypoxaemia) | Action |
|---|---|---|---|---|---|
| Aorto-caval compression | ↓ | ↓ | Normal | Bradycardia/ Prol decels | Left lateral and oxygen |
| Epidural (fall BP) | ↓ | ↓ | Normal | Bradycardia/ Late decels | Left lateral and fluids, raise BP |
| Placental insufficiency | ↓ | ↓ | Normal | Loss accels/ Late decels/ Loss variab | Deliver |
| Abruptio placentae | ↓ | ↓ | Normal | Loss variab/ Late decels/ Bradycardia | Deliver |
| Uterine hyperstimulation | ↓ | ↓ | Normal | Late decels | Tocolysis or deliver |
| Cord compression | Normal | Normal | ↓ | Variable/ Prol decels/ Bradycardia | Monitor pH or deliver |

decelerations with Braxton-Hicks tightenings. This is an indication of severely reduced utero–placental reserve, and labour should be avoided.[20]

### Epidural analgesia

Perfusion of the intervillus space depends upon perfusion from the utero–placental arteries. If the systemic blood pressure falls, then perfusion pressure in the placental bed also falls. There is a well-recognised risk that epidural top-ups can cause a transient fall in blood pressure. Late decelerations, and even short periods of bradycardia, can follow an epidural top-up, and such changes reflect the transient fall in oxygen delivery to the intervillus space. Fluid loading has been shown to reduce the incidence of FHR decelerations. Modern epidural analgesic mixtures also minimise the chance of reducing perfusion pressure, but the risk remains.

### Aorto-caval compression

Supine hypotension also produces late decelerations if contractions are present. If not in labour, then a bradycardia may occur. Perfusion of the utero–placental arteries falls and less oxygen is delivered to the intervillus space. If this reservoir of oxygen is already reduced, either by unrecognised placental insufficiency or uterine activity, then the effect of maternal hypotension is greater. A bradycardia suggests a greater fall in blood pressure. Alternatively, a bradycardia could be viewed as indicative of a greater degree of utero–placental insufficiency. Interpretation should indicate a reduction in utero–placental reserve.

## Umbilical cord compression

It has been suggested that up to 30% of labours may have variable FHR decelerations as a result of compression of the umbilical cord. If the cord is around the fetal neck, then compression may occur between the uterus and the fetal neck. As the fetus moves into the pelvis, it becomes more likely that compression between the fetal neck and the pelvis can also occur. In fact, once full dilatation has been reached, risk for cord compression becomes maximal as the fetal head fully enters the pelvis and as the cervix becomes fully dilated and slips back over the head to the neck! Oligohydramnios and rupture of the membranes also predispose to cord compression.

Compression of the umbilical vein causes a fairly abrupt fall in venous return to the fetal heart. The fall in fetal blood oxygen content is sensed by the chemoreceptors and the FHR drops abruptly. Once the cord compression is relieved, then the FHR rapidly returns to a normal rate. Cord compression decelerations are variable and do not necessarily occur with every contraction. They may be short or prolonged, and may be shallow or deep. Their size is a reflection of the degree of compression of the cord. The larger the deceleration, the greater the interruption of oxygen delivery. As the second stage approaches the risk of unrelieved compression increases. An FHR bradycardia that does not recover is an indication for urgent delivery.

The baseline between decelerations gives some idea of how the fetus is coping. If the baseline remains unchanged, and particularly if accelerations remain present, then the development of fetal acidaemia is unlikely. Accelerations may be interrupted by compression of the cord thus giving the appearance of shoulders (see Fig. 1.3). If fetal catecholamines are released during the transient hypoxia, then the decelerations may be followed by a transient tachycardia. If the baseline rises, then the fetus may be becoming hypoxaemic. It is of some concern that, in animal experiments, repeated partial occlusion of the cord can cause severe brain damage without systemic acidaemia. This probably reflects an effect on the fetal circulation and blood pressure, indicating the importance of cerebral perfusion.[31]

## Rupture of the uterus

If the uterus ruptures during labour, then the FHR appearance is similar to that of an abruption. Initially, uterine retraction will occlude perfusion into the intervillus space. This will be seen as late decelerations. Increasing hypoxia will produce a fetal bradycardia with decreasing variability.

## Fetal behaviour

The biggest effect on FHR variability is the fetal rest-activity cycle.[1] During fetal quiescence, the variability can be quite low. In the absence of fetal movements, it is unlikely that FHR accelerations will be present. Waiting at least 40 min is reasonable in the absence of any other indication to deliver. If low FHR variability persists more that 1 h, then the possibility of chronic fetal hypoxia needs to be considered. Fetal movements cause FHR accelerations and can often be seen during labour. FHR accelerations at any time during labour strongly indicate a normal fetal pH.[32] Fetal movements without accelerations is a situation that should raise concern about placental function and the possibility of chronic hypoxia.

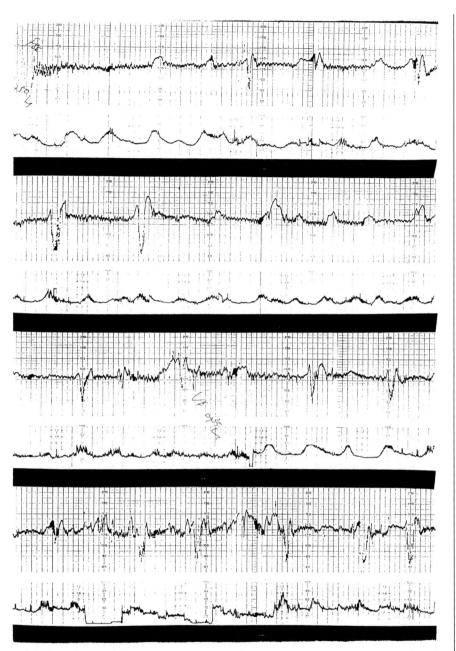

**Fig. 1.3** A continuous CTG at 1 cm/min during labour at term indicating umbilical cord compression without fetal compromise. Note the FHR accelerations were sometimes interrupted by the intermittent variable decelerations. FHR and variability remained normal. The only risk in such a case is of unrelieved compression in the second stage.

## FETAL BLOOD SAMPLING

In a number of cases, the FHR cannot be safely interpreted during labour. A tachycardia suggests fetal adrenal stimulation and suggests significant hypoxaemia. However, fetal tolerance of intrapartum events, especially in the absence of FHR accelerations, requires fetal blood sampling to exclude the development of significant acidaemia. A fetal capillary blood pH of 7.20 or less is accepted as the cut-off indicating a need for delivery. Many FHR changes can occur for various periods of time without the development of acidaemia, and the need for pH analysis is accepted as necessary if operative intervention on the basis of CTG changes is to be minimised.[21]

Repeat sampling is required to obtain an idea of the rate of change of pH and, thereby, predict the possible need for intervention before delivery is likely. The rate of fall in pH reflects placental function and fetal response to perfusion between contractions. The greater the interference with oxygen delivery, the faster the fall in pH. If the FHR indicates significant interruption of oxygen delivery, particularly in a high risk situation, then delivery may be a better option than repeating the fetal blood pH analysis.

## OUTCOME MEASURES

The recent report of the *Confidential Enquiries into Stillbirths and Deaths in Infancy* has highlighted perceived deficiencies in standards of CTG interpretation during labour. Most cases are still considered to have avoidable factors associated with them.[33] The major problem with all studies of FHR monitoring has been the small numbers. Attempts to understand the influence of continuous FHR monitoring on cerebral damage have been less successful and it is not clear whether use of the CTG can reduce the likelihood of cerebral palsy. Using the FIGO classification,[34] cases of neonatal encephalopathy were found to have twice the likelihood of an abnormal CTG during labour.[35] This is mainly in the form of absent accelerations and low variability. The randomised trials suggest benefit in the form of reduced hypoxia,[30] but many fetuses are delivered with umbilical artery pH value below 7.20. A statistical relationship between fetal acidaemia at birth and adverse neurodevelopmental outcome is evident only when the pH is less than 7.05.[36] Caesarean section rate are approaching 20% and yet intrapartum deaths and birth asphyxia causing cerebral palsy together still occur in far less than 0.5% of cases in most units.

## CONCLUSIONS

Whether better training in CTG interpretation will improve outcomes remains to be seen. What is clear at this time is that use of continuous FHR monitoring remains popular and widespread. Therefore, the need for a physiological understanding of FHR changes seems evident as the best way forward. Only when changes seen on the CTG are fully understood can the question of clinical value be appropriately addressed.

### References

1 Spencer JAD, Johnson P. Fetal heart rate variability changes and fetal behavioural cycles during labour. Br J Obstet Gynaecol 1986; 93: 314–321

# Key points for clinical practice

- A CTG is indicated when there is concern about fetal oxygenation

- The tocograph can identify fetal and maternal movements in addition to uterine activity

- The ultrasound transducer identifies regular movements and may display the maternal heart rate from arterial pulsations in the abdomen

- The fetal heart rate changes when oxygen delivery to the fetus is interrupted

- Oxygen delivery to the fetus depends upon utero–placental perfusion into the intervillous space and venous return in the umbilical vein

- The healthy fetus responds to an acute interruption in oxygen delivery with a fetal heart rate deceleration stimulated by the chemoreceptors

- Utero–placental perfusion of the intervillous space is acutely reduced by uterine contractions and during maternal hypotension

- Utero–placental perfusion of the intervillous space is chronically reduced with placental insufficiency

- Fetal hypoxaemia and acidaemia occurs gradually with placental insufficiency; the fetal heart rate remains normal due to raised catecholamines

- Placental insufficiency produces late decelerations with Braxton-Hicks tightenings, and reduces fetal tolerance to labour

- Late fetal heart rate decelerations in labour indicate hypoxaemia of the intervillous space

- Variable fetal heart rate decelerations in labour occur with compression of the umbilical cord

- The most common reason for reduced fetal heart rate variability in labour is fetal sleep (quiet state)

- Fetal heart rate accelerations in labour strongly indicate the absence of acidaemia

- Fetal blood sampling is required when the fetal heart rate cannot be safely interpreted

2  Helfand M, Marton K, Ueland K. Factors involved in the interpretation of fetal monitor tracings. Am J Obstet Gynecol 1985; 151: 737–744

3  Cibils LA. On intrapartum fetal monitoring. Am J Obstet Gynecol 1996; 174: 1382–1389

4  Boehm FH, Fields LM, Hutchison JM, Bowen AW, Vaughn WK. The indirectly obtained fetal heart rate: comparison of first- and second-generation electronic fetal monitors. Am J Obstet Gynecol 1986; 155: 10–14

5  Divon MY, Torres FP, Yeh S-Y, Paul R. Autocorrelation techniques in fetal monitoring. Am J Obstet Gynecol 1985; 151: 2–6

6   Westgate J, Harris M, Curnow JSH, Greene KR. Plymouth randomised trial of cardiotocography only versus ST waveform plus cardiotocography for intrapartum monitoring in 2400 cases. Am J Obstet Gynecol 1993; 169: 1151–1160

7   Khong TY, DeWolf F, Robertson WB, Brosens I. Inadequate maternal vascular response to placentation in pregnancies complicated by pre-eclampsia and by small-for-gestational-age infants. Br J Obstet Gynaecol 1986; 93: 1049–1059

8   Creasy RK, Barrett CK, DeSwiet M, Kahanpaa KV, Rudolph AM. Experimental intrauterine growth retardation in the sheep. Am J Obstet Gynecol 1972; 112: 566–573

9   Robinson JS, Kingston EJ, Jones CT, Thorburn GD. Studies on experimental growth retardation in sheep. The effect of removal of endometrial caruncles on fetal size and metabolism. J Dev Physiol 1979; 1: 379–398

10  Itskovitz J, LaGamma EF, Rudolf AM. The effect of reducing umbilical blood flow on fetal oxygenation. Am J Obstet Gynecol 1983; 145: 813–818

11  Borell U, Fernstrom I, Ohlson L, Wiqvist N. Influence of uterine contractions on the uteroplacental blood flow at term. Am J Obstet Gynecol 1963; 93: 44–57

12  Giussani DA, Spencer JAD, Moore PJ, Bennet L, Hanson MA. Afferent and efferent components of the cardiovascular reflex responses to acute hypoxia in term fetal sheep. J Physiol 1993; 461: 431–449

13  Bocking AD, White S, Gagnon R, Hansford H. Effect of prolonged hypoxaemia on fetal heart rate accelerations and decelerations in sheep. Am J Obstet Gynecol 1989; 161: 722–727

14  Bocking AD, Gagnon R, White SE, Homan J, Milne KM, Richardson BS. Circulatory responses to prolonged hypoxemia in fetal sheep. Am J Obstet Gynecol 1988; 159: 1418–1424

15  Gu W, Jones CT, Parer JT. Metabolic and cardiovascular effects on fetal sheep of sustained reduction of uterine blood flow. J Physiol 1985; 368: 109–129

16  Snijders RJM, Ribbert LSM, Visser GHA, Mulder EJH. Numeric analysis of heart rate variation in intrauterine growth-retarded fetuses: a longitudinal study. J Obstet Gynecol 1992; 166: 22–27

17  Robinson JS, Kingston EJ, Jones CT, Thorburn GD. Studies on experimental growth retardation in sheep. The effect of removal of endometrial caruncles on fetal size and metabolism. J Dev Physiol 1979; 1: 379–398

18  Pearson JF, Weaver JB. A six-point scoring system for antenatal cardiotocographs. Br J Obstet Gynaecol 1978; 85: 321–327

19  Visser GHA, Redman CWG, Huisjes HJ, Turnbull AC. Nonstressed antepartum heart rate monitoring: implications of decelerations after spontaneous contractions. Am J Obstet Gynecol 1980; 138: 429–435

20  Beischer NA, Drew JH, Ashton PW et al. Quality of survival of infants with critical fetal reserve detected by antenatal cardiotocography. Am J Obstet Gynecol 1983; 146: 662–670

21  Spencer JAD, Ward RHT. Recommendations arising from the 26th RCOG study group: intrapartum fetal surveillance. In: Spencer JAD, Ward RHT (eds) Intrapartum Fetal Surveillance. London: RCOG Press, 1993; 387–393

22  Spencer JAD. Fetal response to labour. In: Spencer JAD, Ward RHT (eds) Intrapartum Fetal Surveillance. London: RCOG Press, 1993; 17–33

23  Ingemarsson I, Arulkumaran S, Ingemarsson E, TambyRaja RL, Ratnam SS. Admission test: a screening test for fetal distress in labor. Am J Obstet Gynecol 1986; 68: 800–806

24  Chang TC, Robson SC, Spencer JAD, Gallivan S. Identification of fetal growth retardation: comparison of Doppler waveform indices and serial ultrasound measurements of abdominal circumference and fetal weight. Obstet Gynecol 1993; 82: 230–236

25  Visser GHA, Bekedam DJ. Monitoring the growth retarded fetus. In: Spencer JAD. (ed) Fetal Monitoring. Oxford: Oxford University Press, 1991: 112–117

26  Pazos R, Vuolo K, Aladjem S, Lueck J, Anderson C. Association of spontaneous fetal heart rate decelerations during antepartum nonstress testing and intrauterine growth retardation. Am J Obstet Gynecol 1982; 144: 574–577

27  Grant AM, Elbourne DR, Valentin L, Alexander S. Routine fetal movements counting and risk of antepartum late death in normally formed singletons. Lancet 1989; ii: 345–359

28 Grant A, Mohide P. Screening and diagnostic tests in antenatal care. In: Enkin M, Chalmers I. (eds) Effectiveness and Satisfaction in Antenatal Care. London: Heinemann, 1982; 22–59

29 Wheble AM, Gillmer MDG, Spencer JAD, Sykes GS. Changes in fetal monitoring practice in the UK: 1977–1984. Br J Obstet Gynaecol 1989; 96: 1140–1147

30 Vintzileos AM, Nochimson DJ, Guzman ER, Knuppel RA, Lake M, Schifrin BS. Intrapartum electronic fetal heart rate monitoring versus intermittent auscultation: a meta-analysis. Obstet Gynecol 1995; 85: 149–155

31 Clapp JF, Peress NS, Wesley M, Mann LI. Brain damage after intermittent partial cord occlusion in the chronically instrumented fetal lamb. Am J Obstet Gynecol 1988; 159: 504–509

32 Spencer JAD. Predictive value of a fetal heart rate acceleration at the time of fetal blood sampling in labour. J Perinat Med 1991; 19: 207–215

33 Maternal and Child Health Consortium. Confidential enquiry into stillbirths and deaths in infancy: 4th annual report. London: Department of Health, 1997

34 FIGO News. Guidelines for the use of fetal monitoring. Int J Gynaecol Obstet 1987; 25: 159–167

35 Spencer JAD, Badawi N, Burton P, Keogh J, Pemberton P, Stanley F. The intrapartum CTG prior to neonatal encephalopathy at term: a case-control study. Br J Obstet Gynaecol 1997; 104: 25–28

36 Fee SC, Malee K, Deddish R, Minogue JP, Socol ML. Severe acidosis and subsequent neurologic status. Am J Obstet Gynecol 1990; 162: 802–806

Cardiotocographic assessment of fetal well-being in late pregnancy and labour

*Bridgette Byrne*

# Management of epilepsy in pregnancy

In the 19th Century, Hughlings Jackson, a British neurologist, defined epilepsy as an intermittent derangement of the nervous system presumably due to a sudden, excessive and disorderly electrical discharge of cerebral neurons. The word 'epilepsy' is derived from Greek words meaning 'to seize upon' or 'a taking hold of'. Approximately 1% of the general population is affected and thus it is the commonest neurological disorder that the obstetrician encounters in pregnancy. Epilepsy can be acquired following an insult to the brain (e.g. trauma, infection, or a space-occupying lesion), or may result from a generalised metabolic disorder. However, these cases are few and most epilepsy is idiopathic. Idiopathic epilepsy can be divided into different groups depending on the characteristics of the seizure: (i) generalised seizures, such as tonic-clonic or absence seizures; (ii) partial or focal seizures (which are simple or complex depending on whether there is an associated loss of consciousness); and (iii) special epileptic syndromes, e.g. myoclonic seizures. Seizure activity can be controlled in 66% of patients with anticonvulsant medication. Partial seizures, which are the commonest type of epilepsy in adults, can be effectively controlled by all the standard and newer anticonvulsants. Sodium valproate remains the drug of choice in adults for generalised seizures.

The majority of women with epilepsy who become pregnant have uncomplicated pregnancies and deliver healthy infants. Nonetheless, management issues that need to be addressed in these pregnancies include preconceptual folic acid supplementation, the teratogenicity of anticonvulsant medication, obstetric complications, infant/child care, breast-feeding, contraception and long-term outcome for children of women with epilepsy. Most of the information about epilepsy in pregnancy is from uncontrolled studies and from data obtained prior to the last two decades. A large number of questions remain about optimal management.

Recent recommendations are, therefore, confined to consensus statements of expert groups,[1,2] based on the best available evidence and on developments

**Bridgette Byrne** MD MRCP(I) MRCOG, Lecturer in Obstetrics and Gynaecology, University College Dublin, Coombe Women's Hospital, Dublin 8, Ireland

in pharmacological and surgical therapies. Unfortunately, evidence suggests that optimal standards of care are frequently not achieved in pregnant women,[3] both preconceptually and antenatally, and women with epilepsy do not receive advice about pregnancy.[4,5] Poor communication can exist between the general practitioner, neurologist, obstetrician/gynaecologist and the patient. Sometimes, a woman that has well controlled epilepsy may not have seen a neurologist for many years. To compound these problems, approximately 50% of all pregnancies are unplanned. Thus, reproductive issues should be raised and discussed once the woman with epilepsy becomes sexually active. Optimal pregnancy care involves a multidisciplinary approach. The recent *Confidential Enquiry into Maternal Deaths (1994–1996)* in the UK reported an astounding 19 indirect maternal deaths attributed to epilepsy, a doubling of deaths compared with the previous report.[6]

## IMPLICATIONS FOR THE OFFSPRING OF WOMEN WITH EPILEPSY

The fetal risks include the development of congenital malformation or anomaly and the risk of intra-uterine hypoxia associated with a generalised seizure. Neonatal problems include haemorrhage secondary to coagulation defects induced by anticonvulsant medication, the sedative effects of anticonvulsants in breast milk, withdrawal symptoms in those infants that are bottle fed and the risk of neonatal trauma if maternal seizures occur while caring for the baby. Long-term concerns include the risk of epilepsy and impaired psychomotor and cognitive development in these children.

### FETAL RISKS

#### Congenital malformation

Congenital malformation is defined as a physical defect that results in significant functional disturbance and requires medical or surgical intervention. Observational controlled studies are consistent in reporting that the rate of congenital malformation is increased in women with epilepsy who are taking anticonvulsants (5–6%). The pathogenesis of these malformations may be multifactorial and influenced by exposure of the fetus to anticonvulsant medication or to hypoxia resulting from generalised epileptiform seizures. The role of the fetal genotype in determining susceptibility to these adversities or as an independent contributor to the development of congenital malformation in this group has also to be defined.

Neural tube defect, cardiovascular malformations and cleft lip and palate are the malformations that are most commonly reported in infants of women with epilepsy. The evidence that anticonvulsants are teratogenic is as follows. Congenital malformation rates are higher in women with epilepsy who are taking anticonvulsants compared to women with epilepsy who are not taking medication[7] and the risk increases as the number of anticonvulsants required to control seizures increases.[7–9] A positive correlation between serum drug concentrations in the first trimester and fetal malformation in fetuses exposed to valproic acid has been reported.[10] Certain anticonvulsants have an association with a specific fetal abnormality, for example carbamazepine and sodium valproate increase the risk of neural tube defect by 0.5% and 1%, respectively.[11,12] The profile of fetal abnormality in women with epilepsy appears to be changing. Most of the original studies consist of cohorts prior to 1980 when the older anticonvulsants (i.e. phenobarbitone and phenytoin) were the predominant medications used. Indeed, a retrospective study using the Medical Birth Register of Norway from 1967 to 1992 showed that the incidence of facial cleft declined after 1981 with a concomitant increase in the incidence of neural tube defect.[13] These findings would correlate with the replacement of the older anticonvulsants with carbamazepine and valproic acid. Periconceptual folate, however, may impact on the prevalence of neural tube defect in women with epilepsy taking these medications.

The postulated mechanisms of teratogenicity of the anticonvulsants include an antifolate effect, fetal exposure to toxic anticonvulsant metabolites and genetic susceptibility to the latter. Phenytoin, carbamazepine and the barbiturates impair folic acid absorption and sodium valproate may interfere with the production of folinic acid by inhibiting glutamate formyl transferase. Deficiency of this vitamin has been incriminated in the development of neural tube defect in the general population and the primary or secondary occurrence of this defect can be reduced by periconceptual folate supplementation.[14,15] It is unclear whether folic acid supplementation will reduce the incidence of neural tube defect in women with epilepsy taking carbamazepine or sodium valproate. The pattern of neural tube defect observed with exposure to these medications is different as there is a preponderance of lumbosacral spina bifida and no corresponding increase in anencephaly. The pathogenesis, therefore, of this abnormality may be distinct from that of the general population.[12] An alternative teratogenic mechanism is the accumulation of toxic metabolites. Many of the anticonvulsants are metabolised by the cytochrome P450 liver enzymes to arene oxide metabolites which are postulated to be embryotoxic. Epoxide hydrolase is an enzyme responsible for the detoxification of these metabolites and a deficiency of this enzyme may increase fetal exposure. Prenatal determination of fetal susceptibility to the toxicity of anticonvulsant medications has been performed by measuring the activity of epoxide hydrolase in fetal cells obtained by amniocentesis.[16] Seizure activity or the seizure type do not appear to increase the risk of fetal malformation.[7–10]

## Congenital anomaly

Congenital anomalies consist of minor deviations from normal morphology. Classically, craniofacial abnormalities and hypoplasia and ossification of the distal phalanges were attributed to *in utero* exposure to phenytoin and called the 'fetal hydantoin syndrome'.[18] Recently, these characteristics have been reported with the use of carbamazepine and also in women with untreated epilepsy.[19] Phenytoin was prescribed for conditions other than epilepsy and an increased incidence of facial anomalies was noted in this small sub-group. An interplay between anticonvulsant effects, environmental and genetic factors must occur and there is a large overlap between the described dysmorphisms. Therefore, the term fetal anti-epileptic drug syndrome has been suggested, although the role of hereditary factors remains unclear. Anticonvulsants that are new to the market include lamotrigine, felbamate, topiramate, gabapentin and vigabatrin. Preliminary work with animal models showed teratogenic effects for topiramate and vigabatrin, but results for lamotrigine and gabapentin were more encouraging.[20] These drugs are not approved for use in pregnancy and should be avoided in women of child-bearing age, if possible, until further information about exposure in human pregnancy is available. A register of prenatal exposure to these compounds has been established in the UK.[21]

### The fetal impact of seizure activity

The effect of a grand mal seizure on the fetus is poorly understood. A tonic-clonic seizure usually provokes a transient fetal bradycardia, which probably reflects diminished placental perfusion and maternal hypoxia. Recovery typically occurs within 10–20 min of cessation of the seizure (see Obstetric complications and Fig. 2.1). The rate of congenital malformation does not appear to be related to seizure activity antenatally.[7–10] Increased number of seizures in pregnancy, however, was found to correlate with specific cognitive defects in the offspring at the age of 5 years of women with epilepsy.[22] These defects did not correlate with maternal medications but were also found to correlate with partial seizures and diminished paternal IQ.

### Neonatal complications

Anticonvulsants (carbamazepine, phenytoin, phenobarbitone and primidone) that induce the cytochrome P450 enzyme system in the liver deplete circulating maternal vitamin K and placental transfer of vitamin K to the fetus is compromised. Neonatal haemorrhage (albeit rare) has been documented in infants exposed to these anticonvulsants *in utero*. Specific coagulation studies of cord blood have shown that subclinical deficiency of vitamin K occurs in normal pregnancy, but is greater in women exposed to certain anticonvulsants. These subclinical changes can be reversed by maternal supplementation of vitamin K (10 mg/day) in the final month of pregnancy[23] and, although not of proven clinical benefit, this practice is recommended by some authors.[24] The neonate should also be given vitamin K following delivery.

Most of the anticonvulsants are found in breast milk in concentrations that are safe for the neonate. Phenobarbitone, primidone and ethosuximide can reach concentrations in breast milk that may sedate the infant who should be monitored for signs of poor feeding, lethargy or hypotonia. In some instances, breast-feeding may facilitate controlled neonatal withdrawal from maternal anticonvulsants. Maternal seizures may harm the neonate and, therefore, mothers are advised not to bath the infant alone and to be in a secure position when feeding the baby.

### Long-term fetal outcome

The background risk of developing idiopathic epilepsy in the general population is of the order of 0.5–1%, but this risk is increased 4-fold in the offspring of women with epilepsy. Certain forms of epilepsy are hereditary. For example, certain forms of absence attacks and benign epilepsy of childhood that are characterised by specific electroencephalogram (EEG) patterns have an autosomal dominant pattern of inheritance with incomplete penetrance.[25]

Preconceptual genetic counselling is, therefore, appropriate for some forms of epilepsy. The impact of maternal epilepsy on the long-term development of the offspring has been reviewed by Granstrom and Gaily.[22] Prospective studies have provided conflicting information but, when amalgamated, these children have lower scores in developmental or neurological assessments compared to controls in the first 2 years of life. After 4 years of age, the mean IQ is similar to controls, but the absolute incidence of mental deficiency may be marginally increased. No consistent picture emerges regarding the effect of anticonvulsant medications on long-term development. Specific cognitive dysfunction is more common in the children of women with epilepsy, but this finding also correlates with increased frequency of maternal seizures in pregnancy, partial seizure type and low paternal IQ. Confounding factors, that are often not controlled for, include drug exposure, seizure activity in pregnancy, type of maternal epilepsy, inherited brain disorders and non-optimal psychosocial environment. The comprehensive developmental data which are available pertain to children primarily exposed to the older anticonvulsants *in utero*.

## MATERNAL IMPLICATIONS OF EPILEPSY IN PREGNANCY

The maternal implications of epilepsy include possible increase in frequency of seizure activity, obstetric complications and the toxicity of anticonvulsants, particularly in the postpartum period.

### SEIZURE ACTIVITY DURING PREGNANCY

The primary goal of treatment of women with epilepsy in pregnancy is good seizure control. Seizure activity may increase in pregnancy because of sleep deprivation and poor nutrition. Compliance with medication may be inadequate because of fears of teratogenicity. Serum anticonvulsant levels are altered in pregnancy by haemodilution, altered protein binding, accelerated hepatic metabolism, delayed gastric emptying, nausea and vomiting and poor compliance. As a result, the total level of circulating anticonvulsant is reduced, but free levels tend to increase because of reduced protein binding. Drug dosage may need to be altered in pregnancy, not only to optimise seizure control but also to avoid maternal or fetal toxicity (Table 2.1). Most studies of seizure patterns in pregnancy depend on retrospective data from the preconceptual period. Interestingly, Tomson *et al*[26] recorded seizure frequency from 9 months prior to conception and prospectively throughout the course of pregnancy. Only 15% of women had an increase in seizure frequency and there was no correlation with free anticonvulsant levels. Anticonvulsant toxicity can occur postpartum if the dose of medication has been increased antepartum. Following delivery, medication should be decreased gradually over 6–8 weeks to the preconceptual dose with monitoring of serum levels.

The putative impact of a seizure on the fetus has been discussed above. The maternal risks consist of trauma and socio-economic factors, such as the loss of a driving licence. Status epilepticus is rare and defined as seizure activity that persists for longer than 30 min. It is associated with a maternal and fetal

**Table 2.1** Potential toxic effects of commonly used anticonvulsants

| Medication | Maternal effects | Characteristic potential fetal/neonatal effects |
|---|---|---|
| Carbamazepine | Drowsiness, leukopenia, ataxia, mild hepatotoxicity | Facial dysmorphisms, neural tube defects, hypoplasia of distal phalanges |
| Phenobarbital | Drowsiness, ataxia | Neonatal withdrawal, neonatal coagulopathy |
| Phenytoin | Nystagmus, ataxia, hirsutism, gingival hyperplasia, megaloblastic anaemia | Facial clefting, hypoplasia of distal phalanges, hypertelorism, neonatal coagulopathy |
| Primidone | Drowsiness, ataxia, nausea | Neonatal withdrawal, neonatal coagulopathy |
| Valproic acid | Ataxia, drowsiness, alopecia, Hepatotoxicity, thrombocytopenia | Facial dysmorphisms, neural tube defects |

Reproduced with permission from the American College of Obstetricians and Gynecologists Educational Bulletin Number 231, December 1996.

mortality of 30% and 50%, respectively.[27] When a grand mal seizure occurs, the pregnant woman should be placed in the recovery position and with protection of the airway. Foreign material that may compromise the airway, for example vomitus, should be removed. If seizure activity persists, diazepam (10 mg) can be administered i.v. or rectally. Failure to respond requires specialist input from an anaesthetist and a neurologist. Oxygen should be administered, intravenous access established, and a phenytoin infusion commenced. Fosphenytoin is a water soluble phenytoin prodrug that can be used. Cardiac monitoring and pulse oximetry is commenced and endotracheal intubation and intravenous administration of phenobarbital is required if there is no abatement of seizure activity. General anaesthesia may be administered as a last resort with maintenance of a lateral tilt to avoid venocaval compression.

The old dictum that 'all women who seize after 20 weeks gestation and up to 10 days postpartum have pre-eclampsia until proven otherwise' still applies and magnesium sulphate can prevent further seizures in this situation.[28] However, when pre-eclampsia has been ruled out, the seizure should be investigated fully. A detailed history and neurological examination should be performed. Metabolic investigations include serum glucose, urea and electrolytes, calcium and magnesium. Lumbar puncture may be indicated if infection is suspected. An EEG can be performed safely in pregnancy and the optimal method of imaging of the brain is magnetic resonance imaging (MRI). Fetal exposure to a high electromagnetic field does not appear to have adverse effect in the short-term, but long-term follow-up of exposed fetuses is required. For this reason, MRI is better avoided in the first trimester of pregnancy until further long-term follow-up results are available. CT scan of the brain is considered to be safe with a fetal exposure to 1–2 mrads with abdominal shielding. It must be remembered that meningiomas or arteriovenous malformations can increase in size in pregnancy and other causes of cerebro-vascular disease (such as ischaemia, coagulopathy, arteritis, subarachnoid haemorrhage and cerebral vein thrombosis) need to be excluded.

## MATERNAL MORTALITY

Maternal death is a rare, but catastrophic, complication of epilepsy in pregnancy, and warrants further discussion because the number of maternal deaths reported in the UK from this condition increased from 9 in 1991–1993 to 19 in the 1994–1996.[6] The risk of death was not confined to the woman with poorly controlled epilepsy on multiple medications. Two women had no seizure in the 2 years preceding the pregnancy and one woman presented in pregnancy with two minor seizures. Substandard care was present in 5 cases and related to the health services, the patient and the patients' relatives. Sadly, relatives were not aware of the benefit of placing the woman in the recovery position during and after a seizure and two women were found lying supine with vomitus filling their airways. This report highlights that we should aim to optimise care and provide information to the woman with epilepsy who

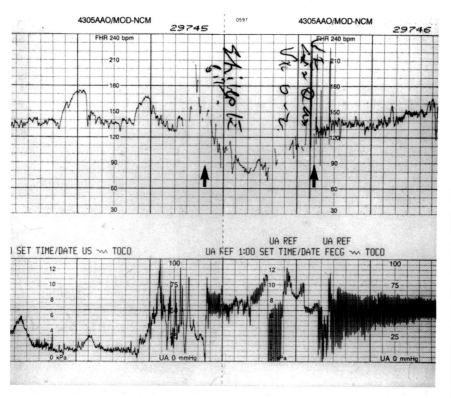

**Fig. 2.1** Cardiotocogram of a woman with epilepsy in labour. The fetal heart rate recording is shown above and the tocogram is shown below. The fetal heart rate and reactivity is normal. The onset of a grand mal seizure is followed shortly by a fetal bradycardia that resolves as the seizure activity abates.

rarely seizes and that simple education of the woman and her relatives may be life-saving.

## OBSTETRIC COMPLICATIONS

Obstetric complications (such as first trimester pregnancy loss, preterm premature rupture of the membranes, preterm labour, antepartum haemorrhage, operative vaginal delivery and Caesarean section) have been reportedly increased in women with epilepsy in some studies, but not in others. The most consistently reported adverse outcome is an increased perinatal mortality. The reasons are unclear, although the incidence may be falling with improved standards of care.[29] Interpretation of the data is hampered by failure to control for anticonvulsant use, seizure activity in pregnancy and socio-economic factors. One in every 100 women with epilepsy seize during labour and this is associated with transient fetal bradycardia which alone is not an indication for delivery. Figure 2.1 shows the cardiotocogram of a multiparous woman with poorly controlled epilepsy in pregnancy who was managed at our hospital and had a tonic clonic seizure during labour. Fetal bradycardia occurs and recovers rapidly with the resolution of the fit and labour continues. However (Fig. 2.2), she had a recurrent seizure followed by a persistent fetal bradycardia, which prompted delivery by Caesarean section. The infants' Apgars were 9 at 1 min and 10 at 5 min and the cord pH was 7.33.

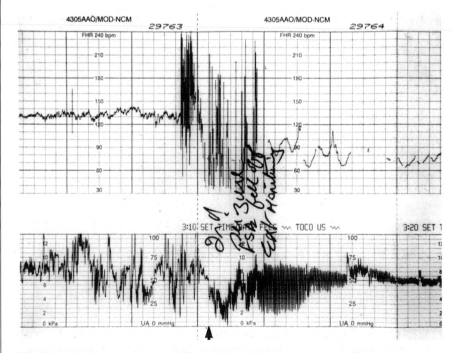

**Fig. 2.2** A further seizure occurs later in labour (see arrow) at 4 cm dilation. This results in a persistent bradycardia. Delivery was by emergency Caesarean section.

# CONTRACEPTION

Carbamazepine, phenytoin, phenobarbital and primidone induce cytochrome P450 enzymes in the liver, increasing sex hormone binding globulin and reducing oestrogen and progesterone levels. For this reason, these anticonvulsants reduce the efficacy of the combined oral contraceptive and the progestogen-only pills. Preparations with a higher oestrogen concentration (50 μg) also have a failure rate that is quadrupled with these medications, but still provide better protection against pregnancy. Barrier methods of contraception or the intra-uterine contraceptive device are, therefore, preferable methods of contraception; if hormonal contraception is chosen, the high dose combined oral contraceptive pill is recommended. No studies are available of the efficacy of depot medroxyprogesterone preparations in women taking anticonvulsants. Sodium valproate, gabapentin, vigabatrin and lamotrigine do not induce the liver cytochrome P450 enzymes and, therefore, do not reduce the efficacy of oral contraceptive pills.

## OPTIMISING PREGNANCY CARE FOR WOMEN WITH EPILEPSY

### PRECONCEPTUAL CARE

The majority of women with epilepsy have an uncomplicated pregnancy and deliver healthy, normal babies. However, the potential adverse fetal and maternal effects of seizure activity in pregnancy should be discussed and these risks generally outweigh the adverse effects of medication (Table 2.1). The necessity for anticonvulsant treatment can be reviewed by a neurologist prior to conception. Gradual withdrawal of medication can be considered if the woman has been free of seizures for a period of 2 years, has had a single type of seizure, and has a normal neurological examination, IQ and EEG.[1] The woman should be informed that the risk of recurrent seizure increases 2–3-fold compared to that if treatment is maintained.[30] Most relapses occur in the first 6 months and it is advisable that treatment be withdrawn gradually 6 months prior to conception; driving is not recommended during that time period.

Conception should also be delayed until seizures are well controlled in the individual who requires medication. This is achieved, if possible, by the lowest dose of a single anticonvulsant agent that is effective for the given form of epilepsy. This recommendation is based on the opinion that all anticonvulsant agents have teratogenic potential and there is no agent that is recognised as optimal for use in women of reproductive age. Fetal exposure can be minimised by divided daily doses or with sustained release preparations where appropriate. Control of seizures with monotherapy is a desirable goal because of the additive teratogenic effect with the risk of fetal anomaly increasing with each additional agent.[6–8] Preconceptual folate (0.4 mg/day) reduces the risk of neural tube defect and should be prescribed for all women planning a pregnancy. Whether the higher dose of 5 mg/day will prevent the neural tube defect associated with carbamazepine or sodium valproate therapy is unknown, but is recommended to those women who have a history of neural tube defect.

**Table 2.2** Recommendations for care of the pregnant woman with epilepsy

---

**Preconception**
  Review necessity for anticonvulsant medication
  Delay conception until epilepsy is well controlled
  Monotherapy is recommended with the lowest dose of the appropriate agent
  Folic acid 0.4 mg/day periconceptually. 5 mg/day for those at high risk of
    neural tube defect
  Discuss risk of fetal malformation or anomaly and the role of prenatal
    diagnosis
  Discuss the risk of epilepsy in the offspring; genetic counselling may be
    required in certain cases

**Antenatal**
  Explain risk of seizures and importance of compliance with medication
  Monitor free drug levels at intervals and adjust according to clinical
    well-being
  Advise good diet, sleep and avoidance of precipitating factors
  Offer prenatal diagnosis
  Vitamin K 10 mg/day in final month of pregnancy
  Multidisciplinary care team with regular antenatal visits

**Postnatal**
  Vitamin K to neonate
  Check for fetal abnormality
  Monitor for neonatal withdrawal
  Breast feeding safe – watch for sedative effects
  Reduce medication to pre-pregnancy dose gradually over 2–3 months
  Avoid sleep deprivation if possible
  Advise about avoidance of seizure related accidents

---

The relationship between epilepsy and congenital anomaly and malformation can be discussed with management plans to diminish this risk. A detailed family history or past history is taken of these defects and the risk of epilepsy in the offspring is discussed.

## ANTENATAL CARE

Neural tube defects can be detected prenatally using maternal serum α-fetoprotein and ultrasound with or without amniocentesis. In high risk populations, nearly all fetuses with open spina bifida can be identified before 20 weeks using ultrasound alone.[31] Cleft lip and palate and congenital cardiac malformations can also be detected antenatally using detailed ultrasound. It is recommended by the American Academy of Neurology that women taking carbamazepine and sodium valproate have serum α-fetoprotein measured at 14–16 weeks' gestation and a detailed ultrasound at 16–20 weeks' gestation. Prenatal determination of fetal susceptibility to the anti-epileptic drug syndrome is experimental at present.[16]

The American Academy of Neurology advise measurement of free anticonvulsant levels preconceptually, at the beginning of each trimester and in the final weeks of gestation.[1] Alteration of the dose of medication should be dictated by the clinical well-being of the patient and levels may need to be checked more frequently if there is poor seizure control, signs of anticonvulsant toxicity or concern regarding compliance. Advice regarding adequate rest, a healthy diet and avoidance of stress cannot be emphasised enough. Family members or partners should be aware of how to manage a seizure and, in particular, be informed of the importance of the recovery position.

Neonatal administration of vitamin K is particularly advised in women with epilepsy who are taking anticonvulsants that induce cytochrome P 450 enzymes and this group would theoretically benefit from the maternal administration of vitamin K (10 mg/day orally) in the last month of pregnancy.[24] Labour should be conducted as normal. Seizure activity in labour is not an indication for delivery unless fetal bradycardia is prolonged or the mother becomes disorientated or confused.

## POSTNATAL CARE

Most anticonvulsants are safe with breast feeding, but infants of mothers taking phenobarbitone, primidone and ethosuximide should be observed for lethargy and poor feeding. Breast feeding may also be of value in facilitating drug withdrawal in these babies. Common sense advice can be of great benefit. Women are encouraged to breast feed in a secure position, for example sitting on the floor with their back supported against a wall, to minimise the effect of a seizure should it occur. The infant should be bathed with a wet sponge and not in water unless another individual is present and, likewise, mothers should not take a bath unattended. Drowning in the bath is a well recognised cause of maternal death and one such death occurred postpartum in the last triennial report.[6] Anticonvulsant dose can be reduced gradually over the first 6–8 weeks postpartum with monitoring for signs of toxicity and free levels of anticonvulsant. Sleep deprivation can be minimised by a supportive partner or family.

## SUMMARY

Women with epilepsy who become pregnant constitute a high-risk group because of the association of the condition with fetal malformation and anomaly and with maternal mortality. Communication between doctor and patient should be improved about the influence of pregnancy on epilepsy and of epilepsy on pregnancy. Preconceptual counselling should begin once these women become sexually active and can be provided by the general practitioner, neurologist or gynaecologist individually or in the setting of a women's health clinic or preconceptual clinic for women with medical conditions that affect reproductive health. Women with epilepsy who become pregnant should be cared for by a multidisciplinary team of general practitioner, neurologist, obstetrician and neonatologist (where appropriate). In this way, efforts can be made to optimise pregnancy outcome. Most recommendations for care, although logical, have not been proven to be of clinical benefit. Proper randomised trials and prospective studies of outcomes will improve our understanding of this difficult area.

## Key points for clinical practice

- Reproductive issues should be discussed with the woman who has epilepsy once she becomes sexually active. Review by a neurologist may be appropriate at this point especially if the patient has been free of seizures for 2 years or more.

- Epilepsy is a cause of maternal mortality. The primary goal of treatment of pregnant women with epilepsy is proper seizure control. Compliance with medication, adequate diet and avoidance of sleep deprivation is paramount. Simple advice, e.g. regarding safety issues for both the mother and child, can be life saving.

- Fetal effects of seizure activity are poorly understood but the risk of generalised seizure is thought to be greater than the risk of anticonvulsant medication.

- The rate of congenital malformation and anomaly is increased in the offspring of women with epilepsy. It may be reduced by use of the lowest possible dose of a single anticonvulsant that is appropriate for the given form of epilepsy. Preconceptual folic acid is recommended and may reduce the risk of neural tube defect in women taking carbamazepine and valproic acid. No single anticonvulsant is deemed to be the agent of choice for the control of seizures for women of reproductive age. The safety of the newer anticonvulsant agents has yet to be determined.

- Seizure frequency increases in approximately 15% of women. Serial measurement of free anticonvulsant levels is advised to monitor compliance and avoid toxicity. Dosage adjustments are usually dictated by clinical well-being. Maternal supplementation of vitamin K in the last month of pregnancy may be of benefit and vitamin K should be administered to the neonate.

- Breast feeding is safe with most anticonvulsants. Enzyme inducing anticonvulsants reduce the efficacy of the combined oral contraceptive pill and progesterone-only pill.

- A new onset seizure after 20 weeks' gestation or within 10 days of delivery is eclampsia until proven otherwise. If this is ruled out (or if the seizure occurs at other times during pregnancy or the puerperium), full investigation of the seizure is warranted.

### References

1 American Academy of Neurology. Practice parameter: management issues for women with epilepsy (summary statement). Quality Standards Subcommittee of the American Academy of Neurology. Neurology 1998; 51: 944–948

2 American College of Obstetricians and Gynecologists. Seizure disorders in pregnancy. Int J Gynecol Obstet 1997; 56: 279–286

3 Seale CG, Morrell MJ, Nelson L, Druzin ML. Analysis of prenatal and gestational care given to women with epilepsy. Neurology 1988; 51: 1039–1045

4 Byrne BM, Sayed S, Turner MJ. Is information given to pregnant women with epilepsy adequate? Epilepsia 1997; 38 (Suppl 3): 266

5 Madden A. Women with epilepsy are not getting pregnancy advice [Letter]. BMJ 1999; 318: 1374

6 Anon. Why mothers die. Report on Confidential Enquiries into Maternal deaths in the United Kingdom 1994–1996. Department of Health, Welsh Office, Scottish Office Department of Health, Department of health and Social Services, Northern Ireland

7 Nakane Y, Okuma T, Takahashi R *et al*. Multi-institutional study on the teratogenicity and fetal toxicity of antiepileptic drugs: a report of a collaborative study group in Japan. Epilepsia 1980; 21: 663–680

8 Lindhout D, Hoppener R, Meinardi H. Teratogenicity of anti-epileptic drug combinations with special emphasis on epoxidation (of carbamazepine). Epilepsia 1984; 25: 77–83

9 Kaneko S, Otani K, Fukushima J *et al*. Teratogenicity of antiepileptic drugs: analysis of possible risk factors. Epilepsia 1988; 29: 459–467

10 Battino D, Binelli S, Caccamo ML *et al*. Malformations in the offspring of 305 epileptic women: a prospective study. Acta Neurol Scand 1992; 85: 204–207

11 Rosa F. Spina bifida in infants of women treated with carbamazepine during pregnancy. N Engl J Med 1991; 324: 674–677

12 Lindhout D, Schmidt D. In utero exposure to valproate and neural tube defects. Lancet 1986; i: 1392–1393

13 King PB, Lie RT, Irgens LM. Spina bifida and cleft lip among newborns of Norwegian women with epilepsy: changes related to the use of anticonvulsants. Am J Public Health 1996; 86: 1454–1456

14 MRC Vitamin Study Research Group. Prevention of neural tube defects: results of the Medical Research Council Vitamin Study. Lancet 1991; 338: 131–137

15 Czeizel AE, Dudas I. Prevention of the first occurrence of neural tube defects by periconceptual vitamin supplementation. N Engl J Med 1992; 327: 1832–1835

16 Buehler BA, Delimont D, VanWaes M, Finnell RH. Prenatal prediction of risk of the fetal hydantoin syndrome. N Engl J Med 1990; 322: 1567–1572

17 Lindhout D, Meinardi H, Meijer WA, Nau H. Antiepileptic drugs and teratogenesis in two consecutive cohorts: changes in prescription policy paralleled by changes in pattern of malformation. Neurology 1992; 42 (Suppl 5): 94–110

18 Hanson JW, Smith DW. The fetal hydantoin syndrome. J Paediatr 1975; 87: 285–290

19 Nulman I, Scolnik D, Chitayat D, Farkas LD, Koren G. Findings in children exposed in utero to phenytoin and carbamazepine monotherapy: independent effects of epilepsy and medications. Am J Med Genet 1997; 68: 18–24.

20 Lindhout D, Omtzigt JGC. Teratogenic effects of antiepileptic drugs: implications for the management of epilepsy in women of childbearing age. Epilepsia 1994; 35 (Suppl 4): 19–28

21 Craig JJ, Morrow JI. New antiepileptic drugs [Letter]. BMJ 1997; 314: 603

22 Granstrom ML, Gaily E. Psychomotor developments in children of mothers with epilepsy, Neurology 1992; 42 (Suppl 5): 144–148

23 Cornelissen M, Steegers-Theunissen R, Kollee L, Eskes T, Motohara K, Monnens L. Supplementation of vitamin K in pregnant women receiving anticonvulsant therapy prevents neonatal vitamin K deficiency. Am J Obstet Gynecol 1993; 168: 884–888

24 Delgado-Escueta AV, Janz D. Consensus guidelines: preconception counselling, management and care of the pregnant woman with epilepsy. Neurology 1992; 42 (Suppl 5): 149–160

25 Adams RD, Victor M, Ropper AH. Principles of Neurology, 6th edn. Wonsiewicz MJ, Navroziv M. (eds) McGraw-Hill, 1997; 329–330

26 Tomson T, Lindbom U, Ekqvist B, Sundqvist A. Epilepsy and pregnancy: a prospective study of seizure control in relation to free and total plasma concentrations of carbamazepine and phenytoin. Epilepsia 1994; 35: 122–130

27 Teramo K, Hiilesmaa VK. Pregnancy and fetal complications in epileptic pregnancies: review of the literature. In: Janz D, Bossi L, Dam M, Helge H, Richens A, Schmidt D (eds) Epilepsy, Pregnancy and the Child. New York: Raven Press, 1982; 53–59

28 Eclampsia Trial Collaborative Group. Which anticonvulsant for women with eclampsia? Evidence from the collaborative eclampsia trial. Lancet 1995; 345: 1455–1463

29 Zahn CA, Morrell MJ, Collins SD, Labiner DM, Yerby MS. Management issues for women with epilepsy. A review of the literature. Neurology 1998; 51: 949–956

30 MRC Antiepileptic Drug Withdrawal Study Group. Randomised study of antiepileptic drug withdrawal in patients in remission. Lancet 1991; 337: 1175–1180

31 Van den Hof MC, Nicolaides KH, Campbell J, Campbell S. Evaluation of the lemon and banana signs in 130 fetuses with open spina bifida. Am J Obstet Gynecol 1990; 162: 322–327

*Ronnie F. Lamont  M. Ruth Mason  Paul E. Adinkra*

# Advances in the use of antibiotics in the prevention of preterm birth

Preterm birth (PTB) is the major cause of perinatal mortality and morbidity in the industrialised world. It is estimated that approximately 13 million PTBs occur world-wide each year, from an incidence of 5.6% in Oceania to 11% in America. In Europe, 5.8% of all births are preterm which represents around 400,000 PTBs annually.[1] Approximately 50% of PTBs occur after 35 weeks' gestation and almost all the mortality and morbidity of PTB occurs before this time. At 24 weeks' gestation, perinatal mortality is nearly 80% and after 30 weeks' gestation mortality falls below 10%.[2] The EPICURE study has shown that 50% of babies born before 26 weeks' gestation will have some form of disability and, in 50% of these, the disability will be severe.

## AETIOLOGY

The aetiology of preterm labour (PTL) is multifactorial with increasing evidence that infection is a possible cause[3] in up to 40% of cases.[4] Preterm labour must be either a physiological process occurring too early in pregnancy or a pathological process as a result of an abnormal signal. The earlier in pregnancy that labour occurs, the more likely this results from a pathological signal such as infection. While the final pathway and physiology, biochemistry, endocrinology and paracrinology of term and preterm labour may be the same, PTB appears to be the result of a heterogeneous group of variables described as the preterm labour syndrome.[5]

Ronnie F. Lamont BSc MD FRCOG, Visiting Reader, Imperial College School of Medicine, London, UK and Consultant, Department of Obstetrics and Gynaecology, Northwick Park Hospital and St Mark's NHS Trust, Watford Road, Harrow, Middlesex HA1 3UJ, UK (for correspondence)

M. Ruth Mason BSc MBChB, Clinical Research Fellow, Department of Obstetrics and Gynaecology, Northwick Park Hospital and St Mark's NHS Trust, Watford Road, Harrow, Middlesex HA1 3UJ, UK

Paul E. Adinkra MBBS, Clinical Research Fellow, Department of Obstetrics and Gynaecology, Northwick Park Hospital and St Mark's NHS Trust, Watford Road, Harrow, Middlesex HA1 3UJ, UK

The interaction of these processes and the resulting insult to the fetomaternal unit is thought to stimulate PTL through a variety of pro-inflammatory mediators such as cytokines, growth factors and bacterial products. Bacteria are known to produce the enzyme phospholipase $A_2$ ($PLA_2$) which is responsible for cleaving arachidonic acid from glycerophospholipids in the cell membrane. Arachidonic acid is the obligate precursor of prostaglandin production and prostaglandins have a key role in the initiation and maintenance of labour. Bacteria also produce enzymes, such as proteases and mucinases, which allow the breakdown of local host defence mechanisms and permit penetration of the cervical mucus plug. Collagenases and elastases produced by bacteria may result in rupture of the fetal membranes and preterm labour. The disruption of the fetal membranes by bacteria may cause release of $PLA_2$ from storage in the intracellular organelles, the lysosomes, and release of arachidonic acid. Finally, endotoxins can stimulate macrophages to produce pro-inflammatory cytokines such as tumour necrosis factor-$\alpha$ and interleukins which may induce labour. Higher levels of prostaglandins and cytokines are found in the amniotic fluid of women in PTL compared to term labour and these concentrations are even higher in the amniotic fluid of those women with intra-amniotic infection who are in preterm labour.[6]

The fetus may also have a role in the initiation of preterm labour. Increased levels of interleukin-6 (IL-6), a pro-inflammatory cytokine which is a marker of systemic fetal inflammatory response, have been found in the umbilical cord blood of the preterm fetus in response to amniotic fluid infection.[7] The elevated fetal serum levels of IL-6 increase the risk of long-term neurological and bronchopulmonary complications. Amniotic fluid infection is associated with an increased incidence of periventricular leucomalacia[7] and broncho-pulmonary dysplasia[8] in the neonate.

Infection is now accepted as a major cause of PTB, particularly very early PTB. When a woman is admitted in preterm labour, irreversible changes in the uterine cervix may negate attempts to stop the process. A more logical approach is to identify women in early pregnancy who are at risk of PTB as a result of abnormal genital tract colonisation. Studies have investigated abnormal genital tract colonisation in early pregnancy as a predictor of PTL and PTB using bacterial vaginosis (BV) or BV-related organisms as a risk factor.

## BACTERIAL VAGINOSIS AND THE PREDICTION OF PRETERM BIRTH

Normal genital tract flora are dominated by *Lactobacillus* spp., which produce lactic acid keeping the vaginal pH below 4.5 so discouraging the growth of other organisms. During pregnancy, the concentration of *Lactobacillus* spp. increases 10-fold as pregnancy progresses. Anaerobic organisms become less common, aerobic organisms remain relatively constant which serves to protect the fetus at birth. As pregnancy progresses, increased levels of lactobacilli make the vaginal ecosystem inhibitory to the growth of many pathogenic or potentially pathogenic organisms, such as *Escherichia coli*. As a result, the genital tract is heavily colonised with more benign flora composed of organisms of low virulence which do not pose a significant risk to the fetus at birth. In BV, lactobacilli are altered resulting in a 1000-fold increase in other organisms, particularly anaerobes, *Mobiluncus* spp. and the genital mycoplasmas.

Anaerobes produce the ketoacid, succinate, which synergistically promotes the growth of other organisms. In addition, the chemotactic response of polymorphonuclear leukocytes and their killing ability are reduced. This results in the genital tract in BV being heavily colonised by large numbers of potentially pathogenic organisms with little cellular host defence response.

Cohort studies from Europe, America and the Far East[10–18] and three case control studies from the US, Sweden and Australia[19–21] have used different methodologies to examine the association between BV or BV-related organisms with the adverse outcome of pregnancy. The studies have focused on PTB or gestational age as an outcome parameter, using different diagnostic screening techniques at varying gestational ages. The majority of these studies showed a statistically significant association between abnormal genital tract colonisation and adverse pregnancy outcome. The degree of risk of PTB was greater the earlier in pregnancy at which the abnormal genital tract colonisation was detected. Screening after 26 weeks' gestation was associated with 1.4–1.9-fold increased risk of PTB,[10,11,15,18] whereas screening in the second trimester was associated with a 2.0–6.9-fold increased risk of PTB.[12–14,16,17] The risk of PTB was almost double for women with BV in early pregnancy (21%) compared to those women who developed the condition later in pregnancy (11%).[16] Using multiple regression analysis, BV diagnosed before 16 weeks' gestation was found to be associated with a 5-fold increased risk of PTB or late miscarriage, independent of recognised risk factors such as previous PTB, black race and smoking.[13]

## USE OF ANTIBIOTICS FOR THE PREVENTION OF PRETERM BIRTH

In four situations, antibiotics may be of benefit in the prevention of PTB: (i) prophylactic use in for women with abnormal genital tract colonisation; (ii) prophylactic use for the prevention of preterm prelabour rupture of the membranes (PPROM) or therapeutically to delay delivery in women following PPROM; (iii) the delay of delivery in women who present in preterm labour; and (iv) prophylactic use for the prevention of PTB or intrapartum chemoprophylaxis for the prevention of early onset group B haemolytic streptococcal (GBS) infection in the neonate.

### ANTIBIOTICS USED PROPHYLACTICALLY FOR WOMEN WITH ABNORMAL GENITAL TRACT COLONISATION

Studies of prophylactic antibiotics in women with abnormal genital tract colonisation have used different methodologies for diagnosing abnormal genital tract colonisation and various antibiotic regimens. The results of all these studies have been conflicting. Some studies[22–27] examined the effects of oral antibiotics and showed no benefit[24,25,27] while others showed statistically significant benefit.[22,23,26] One study was a prospective comparative trial rather than a randomised double-blind placebo controlled trial.[26] Only two published studies used intravaginal antibiotics.[17,28] Both were randomised, placebo-controlled studies of a 7 day course of intravaginal clindamycin cream (CVC) and showed no benefit. However, 100% of the women in one study[17] and 60% in the other[28] were treated after 20 weeks' gestation by which time organisms may have ascended from the vagina into the decidua and be less susceptible to intravaginal antibiotics.

Debate continues as to the best antibiotics, optimum route of administration, and stage of gestation.[29] Due to the 1000-fold increase in intravaginal organisms in BV, antibiotics given directly into the vagina seem logical, but this route may not be effective against organisms already in the decidua, which may require systemic antibiotics. The use of antibiotics as early as possible in pregnancy is rational, since the earlier in gestation abnormal colonisation is detected, the greater the subsequent risk of adverse outcome. In a randomised, double-blind, placebo-controlled, 3 centre study of over 400 women with abnormal genital tract colonisation, a 3 day course of CVC was compared with placebo.[31] This is the largest study of CVC and the most extensive European study to examine the use of prophylactic antibiotics for the prevention of PTB in women with abnormal colonisation in early pregnancy. In contrast to the other two studies of CVC, 100% of women were at or before 20 weeks' gestation at the start of their treatment and 60% were at or before 16 weeks' gestation. Women with BV in early pregnancy who received CVC were significantly less likely (4%) to deliver preterm compared with women in the placebo group (10%). Genital tract colonisation varies according to the degree of abnormality on Gram-stain of vaginal secretions,[30] and the outcome of pregnancy following CVC versus placebo was examined in a subgroup of women in whom the detailed microbiology of the vagina was available. In this subgroup, CVC was most effective when used in those women with the most florid appearance of abnormal genital tract colonisation.[31] The longer abnormal genital tract colonisation remains untreated, the greater the chance of micro-organisms gaining access through the cervix to the decidua and initiating the inflammatory process that may lead to labour. Treatment in pregnancy should, therefore, be early and geared towards those with the most florid manifestation of abnormal genital tract colonisation. While local intravaginal antibiotics have merit if used early in such cases, for maximum benefit combined treatment with systemic antibiotics would be required to cover those organisms already in the decidua.

## ANTIBIOTICS USED PROPHYLACTICALLY OR FOLLOWING PPROM

Most of the extensive literature refers to the therapeutic use of antibiotics following PPROM. McGregor and colleagues have shown that antibiotics used prophylactically for women at high risk of PPROM reduce the incidence.[32] Two recent meta-analyses concluded that antibiotic therapy following PPROM can prolong pregnancy, but was not associated with a reduction in the incidence of perinatal mortality and morbidity.[33,34] These studies were at later gestations where the incidence of respiratory distress syndrome (RDS) and perinatal death is too low to observe benefit. Many studies were conducted at gestational ages as low as 20–23 weeks' gestation which is so close to the limit of viability that a reduction of the incidence of RDS is unlikely. A large, NICHD-funded, multicentre trial of antibiotics between 24–32 weeks' gestation found a significant reduction in perinatal mortality and morbidity, together with a reduction in maternal infectious morbidity and an improvement in latency when these were used in the presence of preterm prelabour rupture of membranes.[35]

## ANTIBIOTICS USED FOR THE DELAY OF DELIVERY IN WOMEN IN PRETERM LABOUR

We are aware of 15 studies in more than 2200 patients, where antibiotics were used in PTL to prolong gestation. In nine of these studies,[36–44] latency was shown with the use of antibiotics in women in PTL and in six studies[45–50] no latency could be shown. In those studies which showed latency, four studies used an antibiotic which was known to be active against anaerobic organisms[39–41,44] compared to only one study[50] which showed no latency.

Newton and colleagues[45] gave women at risk of PTL ampicillin followed by erythromycin, but were unable to find any significant improvement in neonatal mortality and morbidity. They repeated the study using ampicillin with sulbactam or matching placebo, but again no significant improvement was seen with antibiotics.[46] However, women with positive amniotic fluid cultures were eliminated, so it is not surprising that antibiotics were of no benefit since these were discontinued if infection was present; therefore, by definition, antibiotics were only used in women negative for infection. In a large, NICHD-funded, multicentre trial, Romero and colleagues[48] gave women in PTL either intravenous ampicillin or erythromycin followed by oral therapy with amoxycillin or erythromycin, or both, or a matching placebo; they were unable to demonstrate any improvement in latency or reduction in maternal or neonatal morbidity with antibiotic treatment. In this study, only 60% of women completed the trial medication and, despite a power calculation requiring 2000 women to be recruited, only 277 took part in the study. Macdonald and coworkers[24] found no benefit from metronidazole, but based the diagnosis of bacterial vaginosis on culture of *Gardnerella vaginalis* which is not specific for bacterial vaginosis and not sensitive to this particular antibiotic.

Despite the evidence linking intra-uterine infection and preterm labour, no consistent benefit has been found between antibiotic treatment and pregnancy prolongation or reduction of perinatal mortality or morbidity. Many of the trials had a high incidence of post-randomisation exclusions and, consequently, were unable to address adequately the outcome criteria. The lack of consistent benefit may also be explained by the different types of antibiotics used. Agents such as clindamycin and metronidazole are effective against BV-related organisms in contrast to ampicillin and erythromycin, which do not have any activity against anaerobes. While erythromycin may be partially active against BV-related organisms, it cannot be fully activated in the vaginal fluid. The choice of combined therapy raises the question of bacteriostatic and bactericidal antibiotics cancelling out each other's efficacy by their mode of action, together with the problems of trying to carry out large multicentre studies.[50]

## ANTIBIOTICS USED PROPHYLACTICALLY FOR THE PREVENTION OF PTB OR AS INTRAPARTUM CHEMOPROPHYLAXIS FOR THE PREVENTION OF EARLY-ONSET GBS INFECTION IN THE NEONATE

Early-onset GBS infection accounts for 80% of the mortality and morbidity associated with this organism. The Centers for Disease Control and Prevention (CDC) estimated 7600 cases of GBS sepsis, (1.8 per 1000 live births) in the US in 1990 resulting in 310 deaths. In pregnancy, GBS infection can cause chorio-amnionitis, urinary tract infection and asymptomatic bacteriuria and, following delivery, endometritis and wound infection. In the neonate, vertical transmission can result in pneumonia, septicaemia or meningitis.

In 1992, the American Academy of Pediatricians published guidelines for the use of antibiotics in the prevention of early-onset GBS infection in the neonate. These guidelines proved unacceptable to both obstetricians and paediatricians since no specific guidelines were included for women colonised by GBS at term with no risk factors. The guidelines were also lacking in neonatal recommendations relevant to women who had or had not received prophylaxis. Following consultation with the American College of Obstetricians and Gynecologists and the CDC, revised guidelines were published.[51]

The consensus statement supported either a risk-based approach or a screening-based approach to identify those women who should receive intrapartum chemoprophylaxis. The risk-based approach recommended intrapartum chemoprophylaxis to women who presented in labour before 37 weeks' gestation, had an intrapartum fever exceeding 38°C, or had prolonged rupture of membranes beyond 18 h. The screening-based approach emphasised that screening before 35 weeks' gestation was unhelpful, since genital tract carriage of GBS before this time bore little relationship to genital carriage of GBS at term. Screening between 35–37 weeks' gestation was recommended, and intrapartum chemoprophylaxis for all women who presented in labour before 37 weeks' gestation and shown to be colonised by GBS, for women whose GBS status was unknown with a temperature in labour above 38°C, if the membranes were ruptured for more than 18 h or if GBS bacteriuria was present. Irrespective of risk or screening, women with a past obstetric history of invasive GBS disease in pregnancy should receive prophylaxis. The only situation in which urogenital tract GBS should be treated antepartum was in the presence of GBS bacteriuria.

Intrapartum penicillin 4-hourly given intravenously is recommended to reduce the problems of resistant strains of bacteria associated with ampicillin usage. For those women who are allergic to penicillin, a combination of erythromycin and clindamycin should be used. To optimise the yield of screening cultures, the revised guidelines recommended using selective broth media and testing specimens produced from a combination of low vaginal and rectal swabs. In a study to assess the effectiveness and feasibility of the screening-based protocol, the prevalence of early-onset GBS sepsis was found to be 1.16 per 1000 live births prior to institution of the policy, and 0.14 per 1000 live births after the policy was implemented ($P < 0.001$). This represented an 88% reduction in early-onset GBS sepsis.[52]

The relationship between maternal GBS colonisation and the initiation of PTL remains uncertain and the results from clinical trials have been conflicting. A recent study took vaginal cultures from women at 22–26 weeks' gestation and on admission for term delivery, PTL or PPROM. Antibiotics were not given antenatally and no significant difference was found in the rates of PTL or PPROM between women positive and those negative for group B streptococcus.[53] The prevalence of BV in the group was 3.7%, and the number of individuals with lactobacilli-reduced flora was significantly higher in the GBS-positive women. This variation may account for the different findings in the previous studies linking GBS and preterm labour.

## CONCLUSIONS

Spontaneous preterm labour and delivery is associated with infection and is a major cause of perinatal mortality and morbidity. There is good evidence that antibiotics used in women with PPROM can delay delivery, and that intrapartum chemoprophylaxis can significantly reduce neonatal mortality and morbidity caused by GBS sepsis. Uncertainty remains as to whether perinatal mortality and morbidity can be reduced with prophylactic antibiotics in women with abnormal genital tract colonisation in early pregnancy or with therapeutic use in women in preterm labour.

For prophylactic use, better methods of diagnosing and treating bacterial vaginosis are required and more suitable ways of monitoring outcome. For therapeutic use in PTL, antibiotics should be used only for those women with evidence of infection, since only in these women are antibiotics likely to be of benefit.

## Key points for clinical practice

- Preterm delivery is the major cause of death and handicap in the neonate in the industrialised world.

- Infection is a cause of spontaneous preterm labour in up to 40% of cases.

- The use of antibiotics once women are admitted in preterm labour may be too late.

- Antibiotics used should reflect the sensitivities of the likely genital tract flora.

- Bacterial vaginosis in early pregnancy is significantly associated with preterm labour, preterm birth and preterm prelabour rupture of the membranes.

- Antibiotics effective against bacterial vaginosis or bacterial vaginosis-related organisms require agents effective against anaerobes and mycoplasmas, e.g. metronidazole or clindamycin with erythromycin.

- Antibiotics can reduce the incidence of preterm prelabour rupture of the membranes in women at risk.

- Antibiotics given to women with preterm prelabour rupture of the membranes delay delivery and may reduce feto-maternal infectious morbidity. (continued on next page)

- The earlier in pregnancy at which antibiotics are used prophylactically, the more likely there is to be benefit.

- Those women with the greatest imbalance of genital tract flora are most likely to benefit from antibiotics.

- For prophylactic use to be effective, a combination of oral and intravaginal antibiotics may be necessary.

- For therapeutic use, intravenous antibiotics are most likely to be of greatest benefit.

## References

1  Villar J, Ezcurra E J, Gurtner de la Fuente V, Campodonico L. Pre-term delivery syndrome: the unmet need. In: Kierse MJNC. (ed) New Perspectives for the Effective Treatment of Pre-term Labour – an International Consensus. Research and Clinical Forums 1994; 16 :9–38

2  Magowan B A, Bain M, Juszczak E, McInneny K. Neonatal mortality amongst Scottish preterm singleton births (1985–1994). Br J Obstet Gynaecol 1998; 105: 1005–1010

3  Lamont R F, Fisk N M. The role of infection in the pathogenesis of preterm labour. Prog Obstet Gynaecol 1993; 10: 135–158

4  Lettieri L, Vintzileos A M, Rodis J F, Albini S M, Salafia C M. Does 'idiopathic' preterm labor resulting in preterm birth exist? Am J Obstet Gynecol 1993; 168: 1480–1485

5  Romero R, Gomez R, Mazor M, Ghezzi F, Yoon B H. The preterm labour syndrome. In: Elder M G, Lamont R F, Romero R. (eds) Preterm Labour, vol 2. New York: Churchill Livingstone 1997; 29–49

6  Romero R, Yoon B H, Mazor M et al. The diagnostic and prognostic value of amniotic fluid white blood cell count, glucose, interleukin-6, and Gram stain in patients with preterm labor and intact membranes. Am J Obstet Gynecol 1993; 169: 805–816

7  Yoon B H, Romero R, Yang S H et al. Interleukin-6 concentrations in umbilical cord plasma are elevated in neonates with white matter lesions associated with periventricular leucomalacia. Am J Obstet Gynecol 1996; 174: 1433-1440

8  Yoon B H, Romero R, Jun J K et al. Amniotic fluid cytokines (interleukin-6, tumor necrosis factor-α, interleukin-1β and interleukin-8) and the risk for the development of bronchopulmonary dysplasia. Am J Obstet Gynecol 1997; 177: 825–830

9  Chin B M, Lamont R F. The microbiology of preterm labor and delivery. Contemp Rev Obstet Gynaecol 1997; 9: 285–296

10  Hillier S L, Nugent R P, Eschenbach D A et al. Association between bacterial vaginosis and preterm delivery of a low-birth-weight infant. N Engl J Med 1995; 333: 1737–1742

11  Meis P J, Goldenberg R L, Mercer B et al. The Preterm Prediction Study: significance of vaginal infections. NICHD Maternal-fetal Medicine Units Network. Am J Obstet Gynecol 1995; 173: 1231–1235

12  Kurki T, Sivonen A, Renkonen OV, Savia E, Ylkikorkala O. Bacterial vaginosis in early pregnancy and pregnancy outcome. Obstet Gynecol 1992; 80: 173–177

13  Hay P E, Lamont R F, Taylor-Robinson D, Morgan D J, Ison C, Pearson J. Abnormal bacterial colonisation of the genital tract and subsequent preterm delivery and late miscarriage. BMJ 1994; 308: 295–298

14  Gratacos E, Figueras F, Barranco M et al. Spontaneous recovery of bacterial vaginosis during pregnancy is not associated with an improved perinatal outcome. Acta Obstet Gynecol Scand 1998; 77: 37–40

15  Gravett M G, Nelson H P, DeRouen T, Critchlow C, Eschenbach D A, Holmes K K. Independent association of bacterial vaginosis and Chlamydia trachomatis infection with adverse pregnancy outcome. JAMA 1986; 256: 1899–1903

16  Riduan J M, Hillier S L, Utomo B, Wiknjosastro G, Linnan M, Kandun N. Bacterial

vaginosis and prematurity in Indonesia: association in early and late pregnancy. Am J Obstet Gynecol 1993; 169: 175–178

17 McGregor J A, French J I, Jones W et al. Bacterial vaginosis is associated with prematurity and vaginal fluid mucinase and sialidase: results of a controlled trial of topical clindamycin cream. Am J Obstet Gynecol 1994; 170: 1048–1060

18 Wennerholm U B, Holm B, Mattsby-Baltzer I et al. Fetal fibronectin, endotoxin, bacterial vaginosis and cervical length as predictors of preterm birth and neonatal morbidity in twin pregnancies. Br J Obstet Gynaecol 1997; 104: 1398–1404

19 Holst E, Goffeng A R, Andersch B. Bacterial vaginosis and vaginal microorganisms in idiopathic premature labour and association with pregnancy outcome. J Clin Microbiol 1994; 32: 176–186

20 Eschenbach D A, Gravett M G, Chen K C, Hoyme U B, Holmes K K. Bacterial vaginosis during pregnancy. An association with prematurity and postpartum complications. Scand J Urol Nephrol (Suppl) 1984; 86: 213–222

21 McDonald H M, O'Loughlin J A, Jolley P, Vigneswaran R, McDonald P J. Prenatal micro-biological risk factors associated with preterm birth. Br J Obstet Gynaecol 1992; 99: 190–196

22 Morales W J, Schorr S, Albritton J. Effect of metronidazole in patients with preterm birth in preceding pregnancy and bacterial vaginosis: a placebo-controlled double-blind study. Am J Obstet Gynecol 1994; 171: 345–349

23 Hauth J C, Goldenberg R L, Andrews W W, DuBard M B, Copper R L. Reduced incidence of preterm delivery with metronidazole and erythromycin in women with bacterial vaginosis. N Engl J Med 1995; 333: 1732–1736

24 McDonald H M, O'Loughlin J A, Vigneswaran R et al. Impact of metronidazole therapy on preterm birth in women with bacterial vaginosis flora (*Gardnerella vaginalis*): a randomised, placebo controlled trial. Br J Obstet Gynaecol 1997; 104: 1391–1397

25 Carey J C, Klebanoff M A, Hauth J C et al. Metronidazole to prevent preterm delivery in pregnant women with asymptomatic bacterial vaginosis. N Engl J Med 2000; 342: 534–540

26 McGregor J A, French J I, Parker R et al. Prevention of premature birth by screening and treatment of common genital tract infections: results of a prospective controlled evaluation. Am J Obstet Gynecol 1995; 173: 157–167

27 Vermeulen G M, Bruinse H W. Prophylactic administration of clindamycin 2% vaginal cream to reduce the incidence of spontaneous preterm birth in women with an increased recurrence risk: a randomised, placebo-controlled, double-blind trial. Br J Obstet Gynaecol 1999; 106: 652–657

28 Joesoef M R, Hillier S L, Wiknjosastro G et al. Intravaginal clindamycin treatment for bacterial vaginosis: effects on preterm delivery and low birth weight. Am J Obstet Gynecol 1995; 173: 1527–1531

29 Lamont R F. Antibiotics for the prevention of preterm birth [Editorial]. N Engl J Med 2000; 342: 581–583

30 Rosenstein I J, Morgan D J, Sheehan M, Lamont R F, Taylor-Robinson D. Bacterial vaginosis in pregnancy: distribution of bacterial species in different Gram-stain categories of the vaginal flora. J Med Microbiol 1996; 45: 120–126

31 Rosenstein I J, Morgan D J, Sheehan M, Dore C J, Lamont R F, Taylor-Robinson D. Effect of vaginally applied clindamycin on the outcome of pregnancy and on vaginal microbial flora in women with bacterial vaginosis. Infect Dis Obstet Gynecol 2000; In press

32 McGregor J A, Schoonmaker J N, Lunt B D, Lawellin D W. Antibiotic inhibition of bacterially induced fetal membrane weakening. Obstet Gynecol 1990; 76: 124–128

33 Mercer B M, Arheart K L. Antimicrobial therapy in expectant management of preterm premature rupture of membranes. Lancet 1995; 346: 1271–1279

34 Egarter C, Leitich H, Karas H et al. Antibiotic treatment in preterm premature rupture of membranes and neonatal morbidity: a meta-analysis. Am J Obstet Gynecol 1996; 174: 589–597

35 Mercer B M, Miodovnik M, Thurnau G R et al. Antibiotic therapy for reduction of infant morbidity after preterm premature rupture of the membranes. JAMA 1997; 278: 989–995

36 McGregor J A, French J I, Reller L B, Todd J K, Makowski E L. Adjunctive erythromycin treatment for idiopathic preterm labor: results of a randomised, double-blind, placebo-controlled trial. Am J Obstet Gynecol 1986; 154: 98–103

37 Morales W J, Angel J D, O'Brien W F, Knuppel R A, Finazzo M. A randomised study of antibiotic therapy in idiopathic preterm labor. Obstet Gynecol 1988; 72: 829–833

38 Winkler M, Baumann L, Ruckhaberle K E, Schiller E M. Erythromycin therapy for subclinical intrauterine infections in threatened preterm delivery – a preliminary report. J Perinat Med 1988; 16: 253–256

39 McGregor J A, French J I, Seo K. Adjunctive clindamycin therapy for preterm labor: results of a double-blind, placebo-controlled trial. Am J Obstet Gynecol 1991; 165: 867–875

40 Norman K, Pattinson R E, deSouza J, deJong P, Moller G, Kirsten G. Ampicillin and metronidazole treatment in preterm labour: a multicentre, randomised controlled trial. Br J Obstet Gynaecol 1994; 101: 404–408

41 McGregor J A, French J I, Witkin S. Infection and prematurity: evidence-based approaches. Curr Opin Obstet Gynecol 1996; 8: 428–432

42 Nadisaukiene R, Bergstrom S, Kilda A. Ampicillin in the treatment of preterm labor: a randomised, placebo-controlled study. Gynecol Obstet Invest 1996; 41: 89–92

43 Nadisaukiene R, Bergstrom S. Impact of intrapartum intravenous ampicillin on pregnancy outcome in women with preterm labor: a randomised, placebo-controlled study. Gynecol Obstet Invest 1996; 41: 85–88

44 Svare J, Langhoff-Roos J, Andersen L F et al. Ampicillin-metronidazole treatment in idiopathic preterm labour: a randomised controlled multicentre trial. Br J Obstet Gynaecol 1997; 104: 892–897

45 Newton E R, Dinsmoor M J, Gibbs R S. A randomized, blinded, placebo-controlled trial of antibiotics in idiopathic preterm labor. Obstet Gynecol 1989; 74: 562–566

46 Newton E R, Shields L, Redgeway 3rd L E, Berkus M D, Elliot B D. Combination antibiotics and indomethacin in idiopathic preterm labor: a randomized double-blind clinical trial. Am J Obstet Gynecol 1991; 165: 1753–1759

47 McCaul J F, Perry Jr K G, Moore Jr J L, Martin R W, Bucovaz E T, Morrison J C. Adjunctive antibiotic treatment of women with preterm rupture of membranes or preterm labor. Int J Gynaecol Obstet 1992; 38: 19–24

48 Romero R, Sibai B, Caritis S et al. Antibiotic treatment of preterm labor with intact membranes: a multicenter, randomized, double-blinded, placebo-controlled trial. Am J Obstet Gynecol 1993; 169: 764–774

49 Cox S M, Bohman V R, Sherman M L, Leveno K J. Randomized investigation of antimicrobials for the prevention of preterm birth. Am J Obstet Gynecol 1996; 174: 206–210

50 Lamont R F. New approaches in the management of preterm labour of infective aetiology. Br J Obstet Gynaecol 1998; 105: 134–137

51 American Academy of Pediatrics Committee on Infectious Diseases and Committee on Fetus and Newborn. Revised guidelines for prevention of early-onset group B streptococcal (GBS) infection. Pediatrics 1997; 99: 489–496

52 Brozanski B S, Jones J G, Krohn M A, Sweet R L. Effect of a screening-based prevention policy on prevalence of early-onset group B streptococcal sepsis. Obstet Gynecol 2000; 95: 496–501

53 Kubota T. Relationship between maternal group B streptococcal colonization and pregnancy outcome. Obstet Gynecol 1998; 92: 926–930

*Thomas F. Baskett*

# Prediction and management of shoulder dystocia

As operative vaginal delivery of fetal malposition and malpresentation has declined, shoulder dystocia has emerged as one of the more important clinical and medico-legal complications of vaginal delivery. The reported incidence varies from 0.2–1.7% in cephalic vaginal deliveries.[1] The diagnosis of shoulder dystocia is to some extent subjective: hence, the wide range of incidence. The most commonly used definition is failure of the shoulders to deliver spontaneously and/or with gentle downward traction on the fetal head. Perinatal death due to complications of shoulder dystocia is rare, but damage to the infant from associated asphyxia and trauma is not uncommon and carries increasing medico-legal significance.[2]

## PREDICTION

The following predisposing factors have been identified but, in general, lack specificity.

### ANTEPARTUM RISK FACTORS

#### Macrosomia
Macrosomia at birth is the most strongly associated factor and the incidence of shoulder dystocia is proportional to birth weight.[3–5] Many of the other risk factors for shoulder dystocia (such as maternal obesity, prolonged pregnancy, and previous large infant) are those that predispose to macrosomia.

#### Diabetes
Infants of diabetic mothers have a higher incidence of shoulder dystocia

**Thomas F. Baskett** MB FRCS(C) FRCS(Ed) FRCOG, Department of Obstetrics and Gynaecology, Dalhousie University, 5980 University Avenue, Halifax, Nova Scotia B3J 3G9, Canada

compared to non-diabetic infants of the same weight. This is due to a greater shoulder/head circumference ratio because of the insulin-sensitive nature of the tissues that contribute to shoulder girth, compared to brain growth which is not affected by hyperglycaemia and hyperinsulinism.

## Obesity

Maternal obesity has been shown by many authors to be associated with an increased incidence of shoulder dystocia.[3,6,7] Johnson et al found that shoulder dystocia rose from 0.6% in women weighing less than 90 kg to 5% in those weighing more than 113 kg.[8] Much, but not all, of the increased risk of shoulder dystocia with obesity is due to associated factors, such as a higher incidence of gestational diabetes and prolonged pregnancy. Excessive maternal weight gain in pregnancy has also been linked with macrosomia.[4,9]

## Post-term pregnancy

Post-term pregnancy is associated with a higher incidence of macrosomia and shoulder dystocia.[4,10,11] Boyd et al found that the incidence of macrosomia was 12% at 40 weeks' and 21% at 42 weeks' gestation.[4] In the later weeks of pregnancy, the fetal chest and shoulders continue to grow steadily, whereas the biparietal diameter growth slows considerably, increasing the likelihood of an unfavourable shoulder/head circumference ratio.

## Previous shoulder dystocia

In three published series, the risk of recurrent shoulder dystocia ranged from 1.1–13.8%. Expressed as an increased risk of recurrence, the range was 2–16-fold.[5,12,13] Thus, in the vast majority of cases there will not be recurrence of shoulder dystocia.

Most of the antenatal risk factors are interrelated, with fetal macrosomia being the dominant theme. Despite the association of these conditions with shoulder dystocia, the majority of cases occur without risk factors. Furthermore, the predictive value of these risk factors, or combination thereof, is low.[5,14,15] Many of the antenatal risk factors are relatively common, but the condition it is hoped to predict, shoulder dystocia, is not and permanent injury associated with shoulder dystocia is rare. Furthermore, the antenatal prediction of the main risk factor, macrosomia, is unreliable. Hopes that ultrasound measurements would more accurately predict macrosomia have not been born out in practice.[16] Indeed, at higher weights, clinical estimation has been shown to be as accurate as ultrasound.[17,18] In addition, attempts to incorporate shoulder width as a predictor for shoulder dystocia have not been successful.[19]

Because macrosomia is the commonest association with shoulder dystocia and neonatal injury, it has been proposed that elective Caesarean section of fetuses estimated to weigh more than 4500 g, and even 4000 g, should be pursued. However, a recent decision analysis model from the US has shown that for each permanent brachial plexus injury prevented by elective Caesarean section for estimated fetal weight > 4500 g, 3695 Caesarean deliveries would have to be performed at an additional cost of $8.7 million.[20] The futility of such a policy has also been pointed out by others.[5,21] In addition, the majority of cases of shoulder dystocia occur in infants weighing less than 4500 g

## INTRAPARTUM RISK FACTORS

Certain patterns of labour increase the likelihood of shoulder dystocia.

1.  A protracted or arrested active phase of the first stage of labour is associated with an increased incidence of shoulder dystocia.[14,22,23]

2.  Protracted or arrested descent in the second stage of labour is another marker.[5,23]

3.  Assisted mid pelvic delivery carries a higher risk of shoulder dystocia. Benedetti and Gabbe noted shoulder dystocia with 4.6% of mid pelvic deliveries compared to 0.2% in spontaneous deliveries.[22] Similar results were found by Baskett and Allen: 2.8% shoulder dystocia with mid forceps and 0.3% with spontaneous delivery.[5] Thus, while mid pelvic delivery greatly increases the risk of shoulder dystocia, it does not occur in more than 95% of such deliveries.

Overall, the majority of cases of shoulder dystocia have normal progression in labour, and spontaneous or low pelvic assisted delivery. Thus, as with the antepartum markers, the presence or absence of intrapartum risk factors lacks clinical predictive value. Nonetheless, clinical prudence may be guided towards Caesarean section in selected cases with cumulative antepartum and/or intrapartum risk factors.

## MECHANISM

In the fetus at term, the bisacromial diameter is larger than the biparietal diameter. To a degree, the flexibility of the shoulders allows their passage through the pelvis. Normally, as the head passes through the pelvic outlet, the shoulders enter the pelvic brim in the oblique diameter. The posterior shoulder leads via the sacral bay or sacro-sciatic notch, with the anterior shoulder usually accommodated by the obturator foramen. If the bisacromial diameter is large and/or the pelvic brim is more flat than gynaecoid, the anterior shoulder may become impacted behind the pubic symphysis. Usually, the posterior shoulder will descend below the sacral promontory. On very rare occasions, usually associated with assisted mid pelvic delivery, both shoulders may be arrested above the pelvic brim – sometimes known as bilateral shoulder dystocia. The anterior shoulder is more likely to become impacted above the pelvic brim if it attempts to enter the pelvis in the antero-posterior diameter, which is the narrowest of the pelvic inlet.

Once the head has delivered, the uterus contracts down and this causes a reduction or cessation of blood flow to the intervillus space. In addition, the fetal chest is compressed so that adequate respiratory effort is impossible, even though the infant's mouth and nose are delivered. After delivery of the infant's head, it has been shown that the supply of oxygen to the fetus is reduced and the umbilical artery pH falls at a rate of 0.04 units/min.[24] Thus, provided the fetus is not hypoxic up to the delivery of the head, there are probably 4–6 min in which delivery of the infant can be achieved without hypoxic brain damage.

## COMPLICATIONS

### FETAL

Brachial plexus injury is one of the most common fetal complications and occurs, at least temporarily, in 5–15% of neonates after shoulder dystocia. Almost all cases are of the Erb-Duchenne type with involvement of nerve roots C5 and C6.[25] The range of permanent palsy in those infants with brachial plexus injury is 4–32%, but usually less than 10%.[5,26,27]

The most common fracture is of the clavicle, which occurs in about 15% of cases with shoulder dystocia.[28] Fracture of the humerus does occur, but is quite rare. Fractures of the clavicle and humerus heal well with no long-term sequellae when diagnosed and treated appropriately. Fractures of the cervical spine associated with twisting manoeuvres of the infant's head are extremely rare, but can be disastrous.

Provided the fetus is well oxygenated up to the time of the shoulder dystocia there should be, as mentioned above, at least 4–6 min before permanent hypoxic damage is likely. However, if the fetus already has a degree of hypoxic compromise at the time of delivery, permanent damage may occur within a shorter time to delivery. A combination of adverse events, including: traumatic manipulation and obstructed cerebral venous return, along with hypoxia may compound the damage to the fetal brain.[29]

### MATERNAL

Genital tract lacerations are more common and associated with the need for a generous episiotomy and additional manoeuvres required to deliver the shoulders. On rare occasions, uterine rupture may occur in association with vigorous efforts at suprapubic or fundal pressure.

Postpartum haemorrhage is more likely due to a combination of uterine atony, prolonged labour, large infant and increased blood loss from lacerations and extensive episiotomy.

## MANAGEMENT

With shoulder dystocia, the head delivers but does not undergo spontaneous external rotation and recoils tightly against the perineum. Gentle traction on the head downwards and backwards fails to deliver the anterior shoulder. As soon as it is obvious that the normal amount of head traction is unsuccessful, it should be abandoned. The commonest cause of brachial plexus injury is excessive traction on the head and neck. It is essential to realise that the problem lies at the level of the pelvic brim. Therefore, attempts to overcome this by traction or twisting of the infant's head and neck are both illogical and traumatic. Once the problem is recognised, additional personnel should be summoned to provide anaesthesia and neonatal resuscitation. Without further delay, explain the situation to the patient, provide inhalation analgesia, perform a generous episiotomy, and proceed with delivery. The following manoeuvres are available.

# SUPRAPUBIC PRESSURE

This can be applied with the heel of the hand to try and dislodge the shoulder from behind the symphysis. As Rubin pointed out, the adducted diameter is narrower than the abducted diameter of the fetal shoulders.[30] Thus, it is best to apply the suprapubic pressure to the back of the fetal scapula pushing it down and lateral towards the larger oblique and transverse diameters of the pelvic inlet.

## ROTATE THE FETAL SHOULDERS TO THE OBLIQUE DIAMETER OF THE PELVIC BRIM

It is usually not possible to insert the hand or fingers anteriorly and gain access to the shoulder. Attempting to turn the shoulders by rotating the head is traumatic and usually unsuccessful. Therefore, insert the hand or two fingers posteriorly and push the infant's shoulder off the mid-line towards the oblique and transverse diameter. It is logical to try and move the fetal shoulders to the oblique and transverse diameters of the pelvic inlet as these are larger than the antero-posterior diameter.

## MCROBERTS' MANOEUVRE

The maternal hips are hyper-flexed by bringing the knees up beside the chest. As a result, the symphysis rotates superiorly which lifts the fetus and flexes the fetal spine toward the anterior shoulder. This has the effect of pushing the posterior fetal shoulder below the pelvic brim. This is aided by the fact that the McRoberts' position straightens the maternal lumbar lordosis and lumbo-sacral angle, thereby reducing the obstructive effect of the sacral promontory. In addition, the angle of inclination of the pelvis is reduced from approximately 25° to 10°, bringing the plane of the pelvic inlet perpendicular to the maternal expulsion forces.[31] Experimental models have shown that the McRoberts' position reduces shoulder extraction forces and brachial plexus stretching.[32] In addition, clinical experience has shown this manoeuvre is associated with reduced fetal trauma.[5,33] This manoeuvre is strongly recommended as a primary approach to cases of shoulder dystocia.

## WOODS' SCREW MANOEUVRE

In 1943, Woods showed that the relationship between the fetal shoulders and the bony pelvic landmarks (symphysis, sacral promontory and coccyx) was like the threads of a screw.[34] Using wooden models, he demonstrated that fetal shoulders that could not be pulled or pushed through the pelvis could easily be rotated 180° and 'corkscrewed' through without trauma. Using his technique, two fingers are placed on the anterior aspect of the posterior shoulder, using the right hand if the infant's back is on the mother's right, and pressure exerted to rotate the baby 180°. Thus, the posterior shoulder which is below the level of the pelvic brim is screwed around at that level under the pubic arch and can then be delivered from the anterior position. This manoeuvre logically addresses the mechanical relationship between the shoulders and bony pelvis. The principle is similar to that of Løvset's manoeuvre for delivery of extended arms in breech presentation.[35]

## DELIVER THE POSTERIOR ARM

Pass a hand deep into the vagina and sacral hollow, identify the fetal humerus and follow it to the elbow. Flex the elbow, grasp the forearm and hand, and sweep the arm across the fetal chest. With traction on the arm and support of the fetal head, rotate the posterior shoulder 180° to the anterior position and delivery. If necessary, the infant can be rotated back 180° to deliver the formerly anterior, now posterior, shoulder. Delivery of the posterior arm is the manoeuvre most likely to cause fracture of the humerus.

## ALL-FOURS MANOEUVRE

This posture has been assumed intermittently by women during labour since ancient times.[36] One report, based on experience from a farm midwifery centre in Tennessee, suggests it may have application in cases of shoulder dystocia. The technique was originally observed by one of the staff members working with indigenous midwives in Guatemala. In a series of 32 cases of shoulder dystocia, all were resolved by having the mother assume the all-fours position with no neonatal injury.[37] As soon as the shoulder dystocia is recognized, and simpler techniques such as suprapubic pressure and McRoberts' manoeuvre have failed, the patient is guided to the all-fours position on her hands and knees. The theoretical explanation for the success of this manoeuvre is that the flexibility of the sacro-iliac joints may allow a 1–2 cm increase in the sagittal diameter of the pelvic inlet, whereas in the lithotomy position the posterior mobility of the sacrum is restricted. It is also felt that gravity would tend to push the posterior shoulder anteriorly and allow it to move over the sacral promontory. Once in this position, it is the posterior shoulder that is delivered first by gentle head traction. Obviously, getting into this position would be nearly impossible in a patient with epidural analgesia. Although experience with this is limited, it is worth a try if other manoeuvres have failed.

## PARALLEL FORCEPS

Shute has described the use of parallel forceps to grasp the fetal chest and abdomen thereby rotating the shoulders to the optimum diameter of the pelvic inlet.[38] There is limited clinical experience with this procedure, but it remains an option for those familiar with this instrument.

## CLEIDOTOMY

Deliberate fracture or cutting of the clavicle has been advocated to allow greater adduction and narrowing of the fetal shoulders, although this procedure has never been supported by large clinical studies. In practice, it is extremely difficult to either fracture or cut the clavicle in the term fetus. Access to the clavicle is limited and trauma to the underlying subclavian vessels is an additional hazard. Thus, this procedure should really only be considered in a dead fetus or one with a lethal anomaly.

## CEPHALIC REPLACEMENT

Like many unusual procedures, cephalic replacement followed by Caesarean section was born in desperate circumstances when all other methods had failed to deliver a case of shoulder dystocia. Sandberg was first to report that William Zavanelli performed the procedure in 1977 in California, and is hence called the Zavanelli manoeuvre.[39] It would usually only be applicable in those rare cases of bilateral shoulder dystocia when the head has been delivered, but the posterior shoulder has not passed through the pelvic brim and is, therefore, not accessible to the other vaginal manoeuvres. The mechanism of delivery is reversed by grasping the fetal head in the hand, flexing it in the anterior position, and returning it to the vagina. Often uterine relaxation is needed and is most commonly provided by terbutaline or nitroglycerine given intravenously. In many of the cases reported, the manoeuvre has been described as surprisingly easy and followed by a normal fetal heart recording until delivery by Caesarean section. Others report considerable difficulty, even with tocolysis. A registry of cephalic replacement has collated the results on 59 cases, with success in 53.[40] While most of the mothers and infants did well, there was a significant minority with morbidity, including: perinatal death (3), neonatal seizures (4), and permanent Erb-Duchenne palsy (5). In the mothers, two required hysterectomy because of ruptured uterus and 10% were transfused. Another recent publication reported a 92% success rate with the Zavanelli manoeuvre.[41]

Obviously, cephalic replacement and subsequent Caesarean section is a major undertaking and rather intimidating to most obstetricians. However, in those rare cases of bilateral shoulder dystocia in which the other standard manoeuvres are of no avail, earlier rather than late recourse to this manoeuvre may be justified.

Isolated cases of 'abdominal rescue' have been described with failed cephalic replacement. Caesarean section was performed allowing direct manipulation and release of the impacted shoulder through the lower segment incision, with subsequent vaginal delivery.[42]

## SYMPHYSIOTOMY

This procedure has had a long and continuing application in non-industrialised countries for selective cases of cephalo-pelvic disproportion. In cases of shoulder dystocia, symphysiotomy has been proposed, but no published trial is available.[43] Indeed, a recent publication of three cases from the US reported poor infant outcomes and significant maternal morbidity.[44] In practised hands, subcutaneous symphysiotomy can be performed under local anaesthesia within

Prediction and management of shoulder dystocia

5 min. Widespread application for shoulder dystocia would be unlikely, particularly in industrialised countries with little or no experience of the procedure.

Of the many techniques proposed to deal with shoulder dystocia, no single manoeuvre or combination has been proved superior in any trial. The simple and atraumatic manoeuvres should be tried first. It is logical to attempt to rotate the fetal shoulders to the oblique diameter of the pelvic brim as a prelude to all other manoeuvres. This is best achieved by suprapubic pressure and/or the vaginal hand pushing the posterior shoulder off the mid-line. The next manoeuvre, almost concomitantly, should be that of McRoberts. This has the advantage of simplicity, is usually successful in mild-to-moderate cases of shoulder dystocia, and seems to be associated with minimal fetal trauma. When shoulder dystocia is anticipated, it is recommended that the patient should be placed prophylactically in the McRoberts' position.[1] If this fails, the next choice is either Woods' screw manoeuvre, which works well in the hands of those familiar with this technique, or delivery of the posterior arm. The latter direct approach has the advantage of being successful in the vast majority of cases.

If these techniques fail, and it is feasible, then moving the woman to the all-fours position is a reasonable decision. If all the above manoeuvres fail, cephalic replacement and Caesarean section should be considered or, in countries where the procedure is used, symphysiotomy.

Each delivery unit should have a set of guidelines outlining a sequence of manoeuvres for the management of shoulder dystocia. This should be taught and practised regularly, including use of a mannequin, by all staff involved with deliveries. It is reasonable to propose that shoulder dystocia drills should be as important as cardiopulmonary resuscitation (CPR) drills for the mother and neonate. The management of shoulder dystocia will be required almost as often as neonatal resuscitation, and much more frequently than maternal CPR on a labour ward. After a case of shoulder dystocia it is important to document clearly on the hospital chart the type and sequence of manoeuvres used, for clinical audit and potential medico-legal purposes.[2]

## Key points for clinical practice

- Shoulder dystocia cannot be reliably predicted in the antenatal period.

- Clinical estimation of macrosomia is as accurate as ultrasound.

- Elective Caesarean section is not recommended solely on the grounds of suspected macrosomia, as the cost and number of Caesarean sections to prevent one case of permanent injury from shoulder dystocia is high. Furthermore, most cases of shoulder dystocia will not be prevented by this strategy.

- No consistent patterns of labour and/or delivery reliably predict shoulder dystocia.

- Caesarean section for cumulative risk factors in the antenatal and/or intrapartum period may be reasonable on a selective basis.

- All personnel involved with the care of women in labour should be familiar with a logical sequence of manoeuvres to manage shoulder dystocia.

- No evidence is available that any one standard manoeuvre to deal with shoulder dystocia is superior to another. However, rotating the shoulders to the oblique diameter and McRoberts' manoeuvre are easily performed, logical, often successful, and associated with minimal fetal trauma.

- Strong downward traction on the fetal head and neck should be avoided as it is associated with a high rate of brachial plexus injury.

- Shoulder dystocia drills, akin to cardiopulmonary resuscitation drills, are recommended for personnel on labour and delivery units.

- In any case of shoulder dystocia, the hospital chart should clearly document the time and the type and sequence of manoeuvres used to manage the dystocia.

## References

1 O'Leary JA. Shoulder dystocia and birth injury: prevention and treatment. New York: McGraw-Hill, 1992

2 Leigh TH, James CE. Medico-legal commentary: shoulder dystocia. Br J Obstet Gynaecol 1998; 105: 815–817

3 Spellacy WN, Miller MS, Winegar A, Peterson, PQ. Macrosomia – maternal characteristics and infant complications. Obstet Gynecol 1985; 66: 158–162

4 Boyd ME, Usher RH, McLean FH. Fetal macrosomia: prediction, risks, proposed management. Obstet Gynecol 1983; 61: 715–720

5 Baskett TF, Allen AC. Perinatal implications of shoulder dystocia. Obstet Gynecol 1995; 86: 14–17

6 Gross T, Sokol RJ, King KC. Obesity in pregnancy: risks and outcome. Obstet Gynecol 1980; 56: 446–451

7 Garbaciak J, Richter M, Miller S, Barton J. Maternal weight and pregnancy complications. Am J Obstet Gynecol 1985; 152: 238–242

8 Johnson S, Kolberg B, Varner M. Maternal obesity in pregnancy. Surg Gynecol Obstet 1987; 164: 431–435

9 Seidman DS, Ever-Hadani P, Gale R. The effect of maternal weight gain in pregnancy on birth weight. Obstet Gynecol 1989; 74: 240–247

10 Eden RD, Seifert LS, Winegar A, Spellacy WN. Perinatal characteristics of uncomplicated postdate pregnancies. Obstet Gynecol 1987; 69: 296–299

11 Chervenak JL, Divon MY, Hirsch J, Girz BA, Langer O. Macrosomia in the postdate pregnancy: is routine ultrasonographic screening indicated? Am J Obstet Gynecol 1989; 161: 753–756

12 Smith RB, Lane C, Pearson JF. Shoulder dystocia: what happens at the next delivery? Br J Obstet Gynaecol 1994; 101: 713–715

13 Lewis DF, Raymond RC, Perkins MB. Recurrence rate of shoulder dystocia. Am J Obstet Gynecol 1995; 172: 1369–1371

14 Acker DB, Sach BP, Freidman EA. Risk factors for shoulder dystocia in the average-weight infant. Obstet Gynecol 1986; 67: 614–618

15 Sandmire HF. Whither ultrasonic prediction of fetal macrosomia? Obstet Gynecol 1993; 82: 860–862

16 Chauhan SP, Hendricks NW, Megann EF, Morrison JC, Kenney SP, Devoe LD. Limitations of clinical and sonographic estimates of birth weight: experience with 1034 parturitions. Obstet Gynecol 1998; 91: 72–77

17 Delpapa EH, Mueller-Heubach E. Pregnancy outcome following ultrasound diagnosis of macrosomia. Obstet Gynecol 1991; 78: 340–343

18 Sherman DJ, Arieli S, Tovbin J, Siegel G, Caspi E, Bukovsky I. A comparison of clinical and ultrasonic estimation of fetal weight. Obstet Gynecol 1998; 91: 212–217

19 Verspyck E, Goffinet F, Hellot MF, Milliez J, Marpau L. Newborn shoulder width: a prospective study of 2222 consecutive measurements. Br J Obstet Gynaecol 1999; 106: 589–593

20 Rouse DJ, Owen J, Goldenberg RL, Cliver SP. The effectiveness and costs of elective Cesarean section for fetal macrosomia diagnosed by ultrasound. JAMA 1996; 276: 1480–1486

21 Menticoglou SM, Manning FA, Morrison I, Harman CR. Must macrosomic fetuses be delivered by Caesarean section? A review of outcome for 786 babies ≥4500 g. Aust N Z J Obstet Gynaecol 1992; 32: 100–103

22 Bennedetti TJ, Gabbe SG. Shoulder dystocia: a complication of fetal macrosomia and prolonged second stage of labor with mid pelvic delivery. Obstet Gynecol 1978; 52: 526–531

23 Hopwood HG. Shoulder dystocia: fifteen years' experience in a community hospital. Am J Obstet Gynecol 1982; 144: 162–167

24 Wood C, Ng K, Houndslow D, Benning H. Time: an important variable in normal delivery. J Obstet Gynaecol Br Cwlth 1973; 80: 295–298

25 Chauvergus JO, Berg I, Erichs K, Jerre I. Cause and effect of obstetric (neonatal) brachial plexus palsy. Acta Paediatr Scand 1998; 77: 357–364

26 Tan K. Brachial palsy. J Obstet Gynaecol Br Cwlth 1973; 80: 60–62

27 American College of Obstetricians and Gynecologists. Shoulder Dystocia. ACOG Practice Patterns. Washington DC: ACOG, 1997

28 Oppenheim W, Davis A, Growdon W, Dory F, Davlin L. Clavicle fractures in the newborn. Clin Orthop 1990; 250: 176–180

29 Confidential Enquiry into Stillbirths and Deaths in Infancy 5th Annual Report. London. Maternal and Child Health Research Consortium, 1998; 73–79

30 Rubin A. Management of shoulder dystocia. JAMA 1964; 189: 835–837

31 Gonik B, Stringer CA, Held B. An alternative maneuver for management of shoulder dystocia. Am J Obstet Gynecol 1983; 145: 882–884

32 Gonik B, Allen R, Sorab J. Objective evaluation of the shoulder dystocia phenomenon: effects of maternal pelvic orientation on force reduction. Obstet Gynecol 1989; 74: 44–48

33 McFarland MB, Langer O, Piper JM, Berkus MD. Perinatal outcome and the type and number of manoeuvres in shoulder dystocia. Int J Gynecol Obstet 1996; 55: 219–224

34 Woods CE. A principle of physics as applicable to shoulder delivery. Am J Obstet Gynecol 1943; 45: 796–805

35 Løvset J. Shoulder delivery by breech presentation. J Obstet Gynaec Br Emp 1937; 44: 696–701

36 Engleman GJ. Labor among Primitive Peoples. St Louis: JH Chambers, 1882; 40

37 Meenan AL, Gaskin IM, Hunt P, Ball CA. A new (old) maneuver for the management of shoulder dystocia. J Fam Pract 1991; 32: 625–629

38 Shute WB. Management of shoulder dystocia with the Shute parallel forceps. Am J Obstet Gynecol 1962; 84: 936–939

39 Sandberg E. The Zavanelli maneuver: a potentially revolutionary method for the resolution of shoulder dystocia. Am J Obstet Gynecol 1985; 152: 479–484

40 O'Leary J. Cephalic replacement for shoulder dystocia: present status and future role of the Zavanelli maneuver. Obstet Gynecol 1993; 82: 847–850

41 Sandberg EC. Zavanelli maneuver, twelve years of recorded experience. Obstet Gynecol 1999; 93: 312–317

42. O'Leary JA, Cuva A. Abdominal rescue after failed cephalic replacement. Obstet Gynecol 1992; 80: 514–516

43 Hartfield VJ. Symphysiotomy for shoulder dystocia. Am J Obstet Gynecol 1986; 155: 228

44 Goodwin TM, Banks E, Miller LK, Phalen JP. Catastrophic shoulder dystocia and emergency symphysiotomy. Am J Obstet Gynecol 1997; 177: 463–464

*G. Justus Hofmeyr  A. Metin Gülmezoglu*

# New developments in the management of postpartum haemorrhage

Excessive blood loss after childbirth is a major cause of morbidity and mortality in both industrialised[1] and non-industrialised countries.[2,3] In rural communities, where the majority of the world's population live, lack of access to skilled birth attendants who are able to administer parenteral oxytocics, the high incidence of anaemia in pregnancy, non-availability of safe blood transfusion services and lack of refrigeration to store oxytocics worsen the outcome of postpartum haemorrhage. A community-based investigation of causes of maternal mortality in rural Zimbabwe described the leading cause of death as postpartum haemorrhage (40 per 100,000).[4] In industrialised countries, the magnitude of the problem is smaller. Overall rates of maternal mortality in the US are below 10 per 100 000, but of these postpartum haemorrhage is one of the leading causes.[2] In the UK between 1991 and 1993, maternal mortality from postpartum haemorrhage was about 1 per 100 000 births.[5] The difference in absolute mortality rates from postpartum haemorrhage between non-industrialised and industrialised countries underscores the effectiveness of medical care in the reduction of mortality from this cause, and the need to improve this care further, as well as finding low-cost, implementable methods of reducing the problem in environments with limited medical facilities.

This paper will deal with recent developments in the diagnosis, prevention and treatment of postpartum haemorrhage, including approaches which are feasible in under-resourced environments. Emphasis will be placed on the degree of certainty of the evidence concerning these interventions.

**Prof. G. Justus Hofmeyr** MB BCH MRCOG, Director, Effective Care Research Unit, University of the Witwatersrand; Obstetrician/Gynaecologist, Cecilia Makiwane and Frere Hospitals, Private Bag X9047, East London 5200, South Africa (for correspondence)

**Dr A. Metin Gülmezoglu** MD PhD, UNDP/UNFPA/WHO/World Bank Special Programme of Research, Development and Research Training in Human Reproduction, Department of Reproductive Health and Research, World Health Organization, CH-1211 Geneva 27, Switzerland

## ASSESSMENT OF BLOOD LOSS AFTER DELIVERY

The conventional definition of postpartum haemorrhage is arbitrary and clinical, based on visual estimation of blood loss of 500 ml or more. Visual estimation of blood loss after delivery is very subjective, and has been shown to underestimate true blood loss.[6] The use of visual estimation is a drawback in several randomised trials of active management of labour and comparisons of oxytocics referred to below. The wide range of incidence of 'postpartum haemorrhage' in different trials may, in part, be due to differences in the estimation of blood loss.

In order to measure blood loss more objectively in the trials of misoprostol for the prevention of postpartum haemorrhage referred to below, a new method of directly measuring blood loss was recently developed.[7] After delivery of the baby, the amniotic fluid is allowed to drain away, and amniotic fluid-soaked bed-linen is covered with a dry disposable 'linen-saver'. A low profile, wedge-shaped plastic 'fracture bedpan' is slipped under the woman's buttocks and left in place to collect blood loss over the next hour. Blood and clots from the bedpan are decanted into a measuring cylinder and measured. Blood-soaked swabs and linen-savers are weighed, the known dry weight subtracted and the calculated volume added to that from the bedpan. In the WHO trials, this method was simplified by not weighing swabs, but simply adding heavily soaked small swabs to the blood in the measuring cylinder.

In most cases, the great majority of the blood loss is retained in the bedpan, and the method is not unduly uncomfortable for the women. Suturing of perineal trauma is easily achieved with the bedpan in place. Blood soiling of bed linen is greatly reduced. Since the measurement is objective, the method is recommended for use in future studies of postpartum haemorrhage.

Because measured blood loss is considerably greater than that estimated, the clinical threshold for excessive measured blood loss should be set at 1000 ml rather than 500 ml.[8]

## PREVENTION OF POSTPARTUM HAEMORRHAGE

### ACTIVE OR EXPECTANT MANAGEMENT

One of the primary objectives of management of the third stage of labour is prevention of postpartum haemorrhage. In clinical trials where blood loss was measured, the proportion of women losing 1000 ml or more varied between 0–12.5%. In research trials where women are likely to receive close attention and timely standard care, it is not uncommon for women to lose more than 1000 ml. of blood after delivery. In Britain, blood loss above 1000 ml has been reported following 1.3% of deliveries.[9]

Considerable differences of opinion exist regarding the optimal approach to the management of the third stage of labour. Practices vary between countries and between units. Broadly, the approach may be active or expectant.[10–13]

Active management of the third stage of labour is usually implemented as a 'package' including early oxytocic therapy (with delivery of the anterior shoulder or shortly after delivery of the baby), early cord clamping and placental delivery by controlled cord traction following signs of placental separation.

In expectant, conservative or physiological management the above interventions are avoided. Usually signs of placental separation are awaited and the placenta is allowed to deliver spontaneously, aided by maternal effort and sometimes gravity.[14]

Randomised comparisons of active and expectant management have recently been systematically reviewed.[15] Active management of the third stage of labour is associated with meaningful reductions in clinically important outcomes, including postpartum haemorrhage and severe postpartum haemorrhage, postpartum anaemia and the need for blood transfusion during the puerperium, as well as with a reduced risk of prolonged third stage of labour, and a reduction in the use of therapeutic oxytocic drugs. However, adverse effects of active management include an increase in nausea, vomiting, headache and hypertension when ergometrine is used. Manual removal of the placenta and secondary postpartum haemorrhage were more common after active management of the third stage in one trial in which ergometrine was administered intravenously. The increase in manual removal of the placenta was associated with an increased proportion of women in whom the third stage of labour lasted more than 40 min. Neonatal outcomes were similar, but the rate of breast-feeding at hospital discharge and at 6 weeks was higher in the active management group. Other side-effects which have been ascribed to oxytocics administered in the third stage of labour include postpartum eclampsia, intracerebral haemorrhage, myocardial infarction, cardiac arrest, pulmonary oedema and inadvertent administration of the parenteral oxytocic to the neonate causing neonatal convulsion.[15,16] Most of these effects have been attributed to ergot alkaloids which are used either alone or in combination with oxytocin.

## SYNTOMETRINE OR OXYTOCIN?

An important recent development has been the demonstration that the effectiveness of oxytocin in the third stage of labour is dose-dependent. A recent review of randomised trials[17] showed a significant reduction in the risk of postpartum blood loss of 500 ml or more for women receiving the combination drug ergometrine and oxytocin (syntometrine) when compared to oxytocin 5 IU. The advantage was smaller, but still significant, for those receiving the higher oxytocin dose of 10 IU. No statistically significant difference was seen between syntometrine and either 5 IU or 10 IU oxytocin in terms of blood loss of 1000 ml or more, retained placenta and/or manual removal of the placenta, or for blood transfusion. Syntometrine increased the risk of hypertension and vomiting. No significant differences were found in neonatal outcome or the rate of full breast-feeding at the time of discharge from hospital.

There appears, therefore, to be no advantage to the use of syntocinon 5 units. For syntometrine versus syntocinon 10 units intramuscularly, there is a trade-off between greater side-effects and somewhat fewer women with blood loss exceeding 500 ml when using syntometrine. The choice will depend on the relative importance attached to these outcomes. The trade-off between oxytocin

New developments in the management of postpartum haemorrhage and syntometrine use can be summarized in terms of number-needed to treat/harm (NNT). The main results of the review can then be expressed as follows: when 100 women are treated with oxytocin plus ergometrine rather than oxytocin alone, 3 additional episodes of blood loss > 500 ml. will be prevented, while 1 additional case of high blood pressure and 10 additional cases of vomiting will occur.

Oral ergometrine has not proved as effective as parenteral therapy.[18]

## PROSTAGLANDINS OTHER THAN MISOPROSTOL

Prostaglandins have strong uterotonic properties and are used widely in obstetric practice. Prostaglandin preparations are available in injectable, tablet or gel forms according to their intended use. These agents do not cause hypertension, which enables them to be used in hypertensive women. In the management of the third stage of labour, prostaglandins have been used mainly for intractable postpartum haemorrhage as a last resort when other measures fail. To date, the main disadvantages of prostaglandins have been their cost and availability. The main side effects of prostaglandins are nausea, vomiting and diarrhoea.

Systematic review of randomised trials in which intramuscular prostaglandins were used showed modestly decreased blood loss and shorter third stage of labour with prostaglandins when compared to other uterotonics (methylergometrine, oxytocin + ergometrine and oxytocin).[19] Postpartum haemorrhage of 1000 ml or more was also lower in groups receiving prostaglandins, though the numbers were small and the difference not statistically significant. Vomiting, diarrhoea and abdominal pain were more common in the prostaglandin group. One study was stopped prematurely by the supplier because of case reports of coronary spasm and myocardial infarction in women treated with sulprostone and mifepristone.[20]

The results of this review suggest that injectable prostaglandins may be superior to uterotonics in current use in decreasing blood loss after delivery. However, safety data are inadequate to recommend these agents for clinical management.

## MISOPROSTOL

Recently, misoprostol, a prostaglandin E1 analogue used orally for the prevention of peptic ulcer disease, has also been reported for the prevention of postpartum haemorrhage.[21] Misoprostol is affordable, easily stored at room temperature and possesses a shelf-life of several years.[22,23] There is considerable experience with misoprostol use, both for peptic ulcer disease and as a uterotonic in obstetrics and gynaecology, and the drug seems to be generally safe.[24] Misoprostol stimulates the myometrium of the pregnant uterus[25] by selectively binding to EP-2/EP-3 prostanoid receptors[26] and is clinically proven to be a uterotonic agent when administered orally and vaginally for induction of labour.[27-29] Side-effects of oral misoprostol are mainly gastrointestinal and are dose-dependent.[30] Clinically insignificant hypotensive effects of a high oral dose of misoprostol have been documented,[31] a property which can be an advantage over the ergot containing oxytocics which cause blood pressure increase. The uterotonic effect on the postpartum uterus has also been documented.[32]

A major problem associated with the use of oral misoprostol in the third stage of labour has been the occurrence of shivering and pyrexia. Shivering was reported in 62% of women and a mean increase of 0.5°C in body temperature after misoprostol administration when compared to the measurements before delivery.[21] A case of pyrexia of 41.9°C which continued for 3 h after postpartum administration of 800 µg of misoprostol has been reported.[32]

To quantify the side-effects in relation to dosage, the WHO Collaborative Trial of Misoprostol in the Management of the Third Stage of Labour Group conducted a double-blind, double-placebo, randomised comparison of oral misoprostol 600 µg, 400 µg and syntocinon 10 units administered in the third stage of labour. Shivering was more prevalent in the misoprostol 600 µg group and a clear dose-effect relationship was observed (Tables 5.1 & 5.2). Gastro-intestinal side-effects (nausea, vomiting, diarrhoea) were infrequent in all three groups. There were 4 cases of diarrhoea (2.0%) and one case of nausea with 600 µg misoprostol and one case of nausea and vomiting with oxytocin. None of these side-effects occurred with 400 µg misoprostol.

The WHO conducted a large multicentre, international trial in which orally administered misoprostol (600 µg) was compared to oxytocin (10 IU). Post-partum blood loss of 1000 ml was significantly more common in the women who received oral misoprostol. Oxytocin remains the medication of choice for routine prophylaxis. The possible place for misoprostol in addition to conventional oxytocics for the treatment of postpartum haemorrhage requires further study.

An alternative approach is the administration of misoprostol rectally. Miso-prostol (400 µg) administered rectally has been compared with syntometrine for management of the third stage of labour in one randomised trial.[34] Rectal

**Table 5.1** Shivering and pyrexia with misoprostol in the WHO pilot trial

|  | Misoprostol (600 µg) | Misoprostol (400 µg) | Oxytocin (10 IU) |
|---|---|---|---|
| Shivering | 56/199 (28%) | 38/198 (19%) | 25/200 (12.5%) |
| Pyrexia > 38°C | 15/199 (7.5%) | 4/195 (2%) | 6/199 (3%) |

**Table 5.2** Relative risk (RR) with 95% confidence interval (CI) of shivering and pyrexia with misoprostol in the WHO pilot trial

|  | Shivering | | Pyrexia | |
|---|---|---|---|---|
|  | RR | 95% CI | RR | 95% CI |
| Misoprostol (600 µg vs 400 µg) | 1.5 | 1.0–2.1 | 3.7 | 1.3–10.9 |
| Misoprostol (600 µg vs oxytocin 10 IU) | 2.3 | 1.5–3.5 | 2.5 | 1.0–3.6 |
| Misoprostol (400 µg vs oxytocin 10 IU) | 1.54 | 0.96–2.44 | 0.68 | 0.19–2.37 |

misoprostol was shown to be well tolerated. Limitations such as the sample size prevented conclusions being drawn about effectiveness.

Misoprostol (400 µg) administered rectally has also been compared with non-identical placebo in one randomised trial.[35] The mean duration of the third stage of labour was similar. In the misoprostol group, 13/270 women (4.8%) had blood loss of 1000 ml or more, compared to 19/272 women (7%) in the placebo group (RR, 0.69; 95% CI, 0.35–1.37). Of importance was the low rate of side-effects. One woman in each group vomited (both had postpartum haemorrhage). There were no episodes of diarrhoea. Among the last 70 women where shivering was specifically sought as a possible side-effect, 1/34 experienced shivering in the misoprostol group and 4/36 in the placebo group. If rectal misoprostol is confirmed in larger studies to be effective in reducing postpartum blood loss, the low rate of side-effects may be an important advantage of this route of administration. The use of larger dosages may be feasible rectally than are used orally.

## EPISIOTOMY

Bleeding from episiotomies may contribute to postpartum haemorrhage. In one randomised study of routine versus selective episiotomy in which blood loss was evaluated after delivery, significantly less blood loss occurred in women allocated to a restrictive episiotomy policy.[36] Moreover, systematic review of randomised trials shows that the restrictive use of episiotomy is associated with a lower risk of clinical morbidity including posterior perineal trauma (RR, 0.88; 95% CI, 0.84–0.93), need for suturing perineal trauma (RR, 0.74; 95% CI, 0.71–0.77), and healing complications at 7 days (RR, 0.69; 95% CI, 0.56–0.85). No difference was shown in the incidence of major outcomes such as severe vaginal or perineal trauma or in pain, dyspareunia or urinary incontinence. The only disadvantage shown with the restrictive use of episiotomy was an increased risk of anterior vaginal lacerations (RR, 1.40; 95% CI, 1.06–1.85).

Avoidance of unnecessary episiotomies may contribute to the reduction in blood loss after delivery.

## RETAINED PLACENTA

Retained placenta is a potentially life-threatening complication of the third stage of labour. Left untreated, there is a high risk of maternal death from haemorrhage or infection. The current standard management of retained placenta, by manual removal, aims to prevent these problems, but is less than satisfactory. Manual removal usually requires general or regional anaesthesia in hospital. It is an invasive procedure with its own serious complications of haemorrhage, infection or genital tract trauma. Any management simple and safe enough to be performed at the place of delivery which reduced the need for manual removal of placenta could be of major benefit to women world-wide. The injection into the umbilical vein of fluid alone or fluid with a uterotonic drug seems a promising intervention, being simple and apparently safe. The suggested beneficial effect of the umbilical vein injection is that it may reduce the need for manual removal of the placenta by facilitating placental separation.[37]

Umbilical vein injection for the management of retained placenta was first described by Mojon and Asdrubali in 1826.[38] In the early 20th Century, various authors reported on the use of umbilical vein injection of saline solution (0.9%) with volumes that have varied between 200–400 ml.[39,40] Recent studies have concentrated on smaller volumes of umbilical vein injection of 0.9% saline solution with oxytocin, although most of these were uncontrolled.[41-44]

The possible benefits and risks of the use of umbilical vein injection versus expectant management for retained placenta were recently evaluated in a systematic review.[45] The review included comparisons of different uterotonics and fluids administered through the umbilical vein. Twelve trials of variable quality were included. In comparison to expectant management, umbilical vein injection of saline solution alone did not show any significant difference in the rate of manual removal of the placenta. Saline solution plus oxytocin compared to expectant management showed a clinical, but not statistically significant, reduction in manual removal. Saline solution with oxytocin compared to saline solution alone showed a significant reduction in manual removal of the placenta (number needed to treat 10; 95% CI, 6–37). No difference was found in length of third stage of labour, blood loss, haemorrhage, haemoglobin, blood transfusion, curettage, infection, hospital stay, fever, abdominal pain and oxytocin augmentation. Saline solution plus prostaglandin, in comparison to saline solution alone, was associated with a statistically significant lower incidence in manual removal of placenta but no difference in blood loss, fever, abdominal pain, and oxytocin augmentation. No significant differences were found between saline solution plus prostaglandin and saline solution plus oxytocin.

The results indicate that umbilical vein injection of saline solution plus oxytocin appears to reduce the need for manual removal of the placenta. Saline solution alone does not appear be more effective than expectant management. Further research into umbilical vein injection of oxytocin or prostaglandins is warranted. It may be worthwhile to include in the research ultrasound measurement of the myometrial thickness adjacent to the placenta as a method of assessing persistent placental attachment.[46]

## OTHER MEASURES

Other measures aimed at reducing postpartum haemorrhage which have been subjected to evaluation but not shown to be effective include early suckling and nipple stimulation.[47]

## MANAGEMENT OF POSTPARTUM HAEMORRHAGE

### NON-OPERATIVE MEASURES

Postpartum haemorrhage is an acute life-threatening event. An indication of the problems experienced by clinicians faced with its management is given by the multitude of strategies reported, mostly as case reports or uncontrolled series. There is little in the way of systematic evaluation of interventions used in the treatment of postpartum haemorrhage. Essential elements of management of postpartum haemorrhage include: (i) treating shock and correction of hypovolaemia; (ii) ascertaining the origin of the bleeding; (iii) controlling lower genital tract bleeding; (iv) ensuring uterine contraction; and (v) removing the placenta.

Immediate emergency measures include compression of the aorta against the sacral promontory[48] and bimanual uterine compression, the hand in the vagina elevating the uterus to keep the uterine arteries on 'stretch'.[49]

Uterine contraction is usually stimulated by uterine massage and the injection of oxytocin with or without ergometrine intravenously as a bolus injection or oxytocin as a continuous infusion at up to 100 mU/min. When these methods fail, prostaglandin administration is sometimes used. The prostaglandin F2α analogue carboprost has been used as a 250 μg intramuscular injection[50] or by direct intramyometrial injection.[51] Prostaglandin F2α has also been administered intramyometrially. Risks of these methods have not been adequately evaluated. Prostaglandin F2α may be dangerous if inadvertently injected intravenously. In theory, small doses in dilution, injected in several intramyometrial sites after aspiration to check for intravascular position of the needle, may reduce such risks.

Intra-uterine administration of two gemeprost pessaries has also been described.[53]

Rectal administration of a large dose of misoprostol has recently been described in 14 women with postpartum haemorrhage unresponsive to conventional therapy, with apparently good effect, but no control group was included for comparison.[54]

The use of intravenous tranexamic acid has also been reported.[55] It is interesting that this antifibrinolytic agent, for which good evidence of effectiveness for menorrhagia exists, has not been systematically studied in postpartum haemorrhage.

## SURGICAL MEASURES

The usual approach to the management of postpartum haemorrhage unresponsive to non-operative measures is a sequence of surgical procedures of increasing invasiveness. Under general anaesthesia, the woman is examined vaginally to determine the source of bleeding. Good lighting and assistance with broad retractors to retract the vaginal walls are essential. If adequate retractors are not available, obstetric forceps with the curvature facing outwards may be used. If there is active bleeding from tears of the vagina or cervix, it is controlled by placement of haemostatic sutures. If bleeding is from the uterine cavity, manual examination for uterine tears or retained products of conception is carried out. Any retained products of conception are removed manually or with ovum forceps or a large diameter curette. Packing of the uterine cavity with large gauze rolls or abdominal packs has enjoyed a recent resurgence of interest. Alternative methods reported are the use of a Sengstaken-Blakemore tube[56] or a Foley catheter with a large bulb[57] within the uterine cavity. These methods have not to our knowledge been systematically evaluated.

If uterine bleeding continues, defective coagulation should be corrected before laparotomy is performed. If the cause of the bleeding is uterine rupture, this may be repaired, or hysterectomy performed. Blood flow to the uterus may be reduced by ligating the anterior branches of the internal iliac arteries, or step-wise ligation of the uterine and ovarian arteries.[58] When these measures fail, the usual approach has been total or subtotal hysterectomy. Recently, an alternative approach has been suggested.[59] Direct compression of uterine bleeding sites has been achieved in 5 reported cases by means of a 'brace' suture incorporating the full thickness of the intact uterus.

The management of postpartum haemorrhage is an emergency situation which requires swift action and a systematic approach. The various methods used to manage postpartum haemorrhage have not been evaluated by means of randomised trials. There is clearly a need for trials to assess the effectiveness of the various treatment options to allow an evidence-based approach to this most dangerous and terrifying obstetric complication.

## CONCLUSIONS

We have highlighted the evidence from recent systematic reviews of the literature which has established the effectiveness of active management of the third stage of labour in preventing postpartum haemorrhage, and the relative effectiveness and complications of various pharmacological options; the evidence regarding other methods of reducing blood loss after delivery; recent developments in the use of misoprostol for both the prevention and management of postpartum haemorrhage; and the need for further research to determine the effectiveness and optimal dosage and route of administration of misoprostol for the prevention of postpartum haemorrhage. The various strategies used to manage postpartum haemorrhage once it occurs have been reviewed and the surgical treatment.

### Key points for clinical practice

- Postpartum haemorrhage remains a major cause of death.

- Visual estimation underestimates blood loss after delivery.

- A new research method for measurement of postpartum blood loss is described.

- Active management of the third stage of labour reduces postpartum haemorrhage.

- Oxytocin (10 IU) is marginally less effective than syntometrine, with significantly fewer side-effects.

- Misoprostol administered orally postpartum causes dose-dependent shivering and pyrexia.

- The effectiveness of misoprostol in the prevention of postpartum haemorrhage is not yet established. (continued on next page)

- Episiotomy increases blood loss and is often unnecessary.

- Umbilical vein injection may reduce the need for manual removal of the placenta.

- Multiple interventions for the management of postpartum haemorrhage have been described, but not evaluated systematically, e.g. rectal misoprostol and tranexamic acid.

- Stepwise devascularisation of the uterus or a 'brace' suture may avoid the need for hysterectomy.

## References

1 Kwast BE. Postpartum haemorrhage: its contribution to maternal mortality. Midwifery 1991; 7: 64–70

2 Berg CI, Atrash HK, Koonin, LM, Tucker M. Pregnancy-related mortality in the United States, 1987–1990. Obstet Gynecol 1996; 88: 161–167

3 Grimes DA. The morbidity and mortality of pregnancy: still a risky business. Am J Obstet Gynecol 1994; 170: 1489–1494

4 Fawcus S, Mbizvo MT, Lindmark G, Nystrom L, Maternal Mortality Study Group. Community based investigation of causes of maternal mortality in rural and urban Zimbabwe. Cent Afr J Med 1995; 41: 105–113

5 Department of Health, Welsh Office, Scottish Home and Health Department, Department of Health and Social Security. Report of confidential enquiries into maternal deaths in the United Kingdom 1991–1993. London: HMSO, 1996

6 Pritchard JA, Baldwin RM, Dickey JC, Wiggins KM. Blood volume changes in pregnancy and the puerperium. Am J Obstet Gynecol 1962; 84: 172

7 Bamigboye AA, Merrell DA, Hofmeyr GJ, Mitchell R. Randomized comparison of rectal misoprostol with syntometrine for management of third stage of labor. Acta Obstet Gynecol Scand 1998; 77: 178–181

8 Joupilla P. Postpartum haemorrhage. Curr Opin Obstet Gynecol 1995; 7: 446–450

9 Stones RW, Paterson CM, Saunders NStG. Risk factors for major obstetric haemorrhage. Eur J Obstet Gynecol Reprod Biol 1993; 48: 15–18

10 Elbourne D. Care in the third stage of labour. In: Robinson S, Thomson AM. (eds) Midwives, Research and Childbirth, vol 4. London: Chapman & Hall, 1995; 192–207.

11 Gyte G. The significance of blood loss at delivery. MIDIRS Midwifery Dig 1992; 2: 88–92

12 Prendiville WJ. The prevention of post partum haemorrhage: optimising routine management of the third stage of labour. Eur J Obstet Gynecol Reprod Biol 1996; 69: 19–24

13 Prendiville WJ, Elbourne DR. Care during the third stage of labour. In: Chalmers I, Enkin M, Keirse MJNC. (eds) Effective Care in Pregnancy and Childbirth. Oxford: OUP, 1989; 1145–1169

14 Gyte GML. Evaluation of the meta-analyses on the effects, on both mother and baby, of the various components of 'active' management of the third stage of labour. Midwifery 1994; 10: 183–199.

15 Prendiville WJ, Elbourne D, McDonald S. Active versus expectant management of the third stage of labour (Cochrane Review). In: The Cochrane Library, Issue 2. Oxford: Update Software, 1999

16 McDonald SJ, Prendiville WJ, Blair E. Randomised controlled trial of oxytocin alone vs oxytocin and ergometrine in active management of third stage of labour. BMJ 1993; 307: 1167–1171

17 McDonald S, Prendiville WJ, Elbourne D. Prophylactic syntometrine versus oxytocin for delivery of the placenta (Cochrane Review). In: The Cochrane Library, Issue 2. Oxford: Update Software, 1999

18 De Groot ANJA, van Roosmalen J, van Dongen PWJ, Borm GF. A placebo-controlled trial

of oral ergometrine to reduce postpartum hemorrhage. Acta Obstet Gynecol Scand 1996; 75: 464–468

19  Gülmezoglu AM. Prostaglandins for prevention of postpartum haemorrhage (Cochrane Review). In: The Cochrane Library, Issue 2. Oxford: Update Software, 1999

20  Van Selm M, Kanhai HHH, Keirse MJNC. Preventing the recurrence of atonic postpartum haemorrhage, a double-blind trial. Acta Obstet Gynecol Scand, 1995; 74: 270–274

21  El-Refaey H, O'Brien P, Morafa W, Walder J, Rodeck C. Use of oral misoprostol in the prevention of postpartum haemorrhage. Br J Obstet Gynaecol 1997; 104: 336–339

22  Kararli TT, Catalano T, Needham TE, Finnegan PM. Mechanism of misoprostol stabilisation in hydroxypropyl methylcellulose. Adv Exp Med Biol 1991; 302: 275–289

23  Gaud HT, Connors KA. Misoprostol dehydration kinetics in aqueous solution in the presence of hydroxypropyl methylcellulose. J Pharm Sci 1992; 81: 145–148

24  Collins PW. Misoprostol: discovery, development and clinical applications. Med Res Rev 1990; 10: 149–172

25  Norman JE, Thong KJ, Baird DT. Uterine contractility and induction of abortion in early pregnancy by misoprostol and mifepristone. Lancet 1991; 338: 1233–1236

26  Senior J, Marshall K, Sangha R, Clayton JK. In vitro characterisation of prostanoid receptors on human myometrium at term pregnancy. Br J Pharm 1993; 108: 501–506

27  Fletcher H, Mitchell S, Fredrick J, Simeon D, Brown D. Intravaginal misoprostol versus dinoprostone as cervical ripening and labour inducing agents. Obstet Gynecol 1994; 83: 244–247

28  Hofmeyr GJ, Gülmezoglu AM. Vaginal misoprostol for cervical ripening and labour induction in late pregnancy (Cochrane Review). In: The Cochrane Library, Issue 2. Oxford: Update Software, 1999

29  Alfirevic Z, Howarth G, Gausmann A. Oral misoprostol for induction of labour with a viable fetus (Cochrane Review). In: The Cochrane Library, Issue 2. Oxford: Update Software, 1999

30  Inman WHW. Report on current PEM studies: drugs for peptic ulcer or reflux. Prescript Event Monit News 1991; 7: 32–34

31  Brecht T. Effects of misoprostol on human circulation. Prostaglandins 1987; 33 (Suppl): 51–59

32  Chong YS, Chua S, Arulkumaran S. Can oral misoprostol be used as an alternative to parenteral oxytocics in the active management of the third stage of labour? A preliminary study of its effect on the postpartum uterus [Abstract]. The Royal Australian and Royal New Zealand Colleges of Obstetricians and Gynaecologists Combined Scientific Meeting, Brisbane, 28 April–2 May, 1997; 61

33  Lumbiganon P, Hofmeyr GJ, Gülmezoglu AM, Pinol A, Villar J. Misoprostol dose-related shivering and pyrexia in the third stage of labour. Br J Obstet Gynaecol 1999; 106: 304–308

34  Bamigboye AA, Merrell DA, Hofmeyr GJ, Mitchell R. Randomised comparison of rectal misoprostol with syntometrine for management of third stage of labor. Acta Obstet Gynecol Scand 1998; 77: 178–181

35  Bamigboye AA, Hofmeyr GJ, Merrell DA. Rectal misoprostol in the prevention of postpartum hemorrhage: a placebo-controlled trial. Am J Obstet Gynecol 1998; 179: 1043–1046

36  House MJ, Cario G, Jones MH. Episiotomy and the perineum: a random controlled trial. J Obstet Gynaecol 1986; 7: 107–110

37  Carroli G. Management of retained placenta by umbilical vein injection. Br J Obstet Gynaecol 1991; 98: 348–350

38  Koerting W. El metodo de Mojon Gabaston en el tratamiento de las complicaciones del alumbramiento. Semana Med 1926; 33: 353–365

39  Gabaston JA. Eine neue Methode kuenstlicher Plazentaloeung. Muenchener Mediziner Wochenzchrift 1914; 61: 651

40  Jarcho A. Management of retained placenta. Surg Gynecol Obstet 1928; 46: 265–272

41  Neri A, Goldman J, Gans B. Intra-umbilical vein injection of pitocin. A new method in the management of the third stage of labor. Harefuah 1966; 70: 351–353

42  Golan A, Lidor AL, Wexler S, David MP. A new method for the management of the

retained placenta. Am J Obstet Gynecol 1983; 146: 708–709

43  Heinonen PK, Pihkala H. Pharmacologic management and controlled cord traction in the third stage of labour. Ann Chir Gynaecol 1985; 74: 31–35

44  Hauksson A. Oxytocin injection into the umbilical vein in women with retained placenta. A questionable method. Am J Obstet Gynecol 1986; 125: 1140

45  Carroli G, Bergel E. Umbilical vein injection for management of retained placenta (Cochrane Review). In: The Cochrane Library, Issue 2. Oxford: Update Software, 1999

46  Herman A, Weinraub Z, Bukovsky I et al. Dynamic ultrasonographic imaging of the third stage of labor: new perspectives into third-stage mechanisms. Am J Obstet Gynecol 1993; 168: 1496–1499

47  Bullough CHW, Msuku RS, Karonde L. Early suckling and postpartum haemorrhage: controlled trial in deliveries by traditional birth attendants. Lancet 1989; ii: 522–525

48  Roberts WE. Emergency obstetric management of postpartum hemorrhage. Obstet Gynecol Clin North Am 1995; 22: 283–302

49  Drife J. Management of primary postpartum haemorrhage. Br J Obstet Gynaecol 1997; 104: 275–277

50  Merrikay AO, Mariano JP. Controlling refractory postpartum haemorrhage with hemabate sterile solution. Am J Obstet Gynecol 1990; 162: 205–208

51  Bigrigg A, Chui D, Chissell S, Read MD. Use of intramyometrial 15-methyl prostaglandin F2 alpha to control atonic postpartum haemorrhage following vaginal delivery and failure of conventional therapy. Br J Obstet Gynaecol 1991; 98: 734–736

52  Jacobs M, Arias F. Intramyometrial prostaglandin F2 in the treatment of severe postpartum hemorrhage. Obstet Gynecol 1980; 55: 665–666

53  El-Lakany N, Harlow RA. The use of gemeprost pessaries to arrest postpartum haemorrhage. Br J Obstet Gynaecol 1994; 101: 277

54  O'Brien P, El-Refaey H, Gordon A, Geary M, Rodeck CH. Rectally administered misoprostol for the treatment of postpartum hemorrhage unresponsive to oxytocin and ergometrine: a descriptive study. Obstet Gynecol 1998; 92: 212–214

55  Alok KA, Hagen P, Webb JB. Tranexamic acid in the management of postpartum haemorrhage. Br J Obstet Gynaecol 1996; 103: 1250–1251

56  Katesmark M, Brown R, Raju KS. Successful use of a Sengstaken-Blakemore tube to control massive postpartum haemorrhage. Br J Obstet Gynaecol 1994; 101: 259–260

57  Gilstrap LC, Ramin SM. Postpartum hemorrhage. Clin Obstet Gynecol 1994; 37: 824–830

58  AbdRabbo SA. Stepwise uterine devascularisation: a novel technique for management of uncontrollable postpartum haemorrhage with preservation of the uterus. Am J Obstet Gynecol 1994; 171: 694–700

59  B-Lynch C, Coker A, Lawal AH, Abu J, Cowen MJ. The B-Lynch surgical technique for the control of massive postpartum haemorrhage: an alternative to hysterectomy? Five cases reported. Br J Obstet Gynaecol 1997; 104: 372–375

*Shirley A. Steel*

# Risk management in obstetrical practice

Clinical risk management can be described as 'a particular approach to improving quality of care which places special emphasis on occasions in which patients are harmed or disturbed by their treatment'.[1] The aim, therefore, of clinical risk management is to reduce harm and the occurrence of preventable adverse effects. This can be achieved in two ways. In the first place, steps may be possible to prevent an incident happening, although the sequence of events that may contribute to an incident cannot always be foreseen. Furthermore, it is virtually impossible to assess or measure what may have been prevented. Secondly, steps may be taken to prevent a recurrence of an incident after it has occurred.

Risk management can, therefore, be seen as the identification, analysis and control of risks. The clinical risk management strategy of Peterborough Hospitals NHS Trust is 'to ensure the highest possible quality of care, that patients are treated in a safe environment and subjected to the minimum risk'. Quality may be defined as doing the right things at the right time, and the first time.[2] Clinical risk management is not, however, a discrete entity. Almost every aspect of obstetrical practice has some impact on clinical risk. Work undertaken in audit and education and clinical governance, for example, are very closely intertwined with clinical risk management.

Communication plays a central role in risk management and, therefore, quality of care. The communication of the event of a clinical incident to the necessary professionals, the communication between doctors at the time of handing over of care, the communication between a trainee and a consultant over the telephone at night, and the communications between health professionals and their patients are crucially important in reducing the chance of adverse events. This single factor is cited regularly as a major contributory factor in examples of substandard care in the confidential enquiries. Poor communication is also a major source of patient complaint and litigation.

**Shirley A. Steel** MB BS FRCOG, Consultant Obstetrician and Gynaecologist, Peterborough District Hospital, Peterborough Hospitals NHS Trust, Thorpe Road, Peterborough PE3 6DA, UK

## CLINICAL INCIDENTS

One of the first steps in recognising the occurrence of adverse outcome or harm to patients is to acquire information regarding clinical incidents. The term 'clinical' rather than 'critical' is preferable since 'critical' could be misconstrued as a pejorative term, even though it is noted that the final bulletin from the RCOG Clinical Audit Unit has adopted the term 'critical'.[3] Many doctors express initial reluctance at instituting a method of reporting of clinical incidents. This is often related to justifiable concerns regarding the available clinical time to deal with such reports. Doctors and other health professionals may also have concerns that, by reporting cases, they may themselves be subjected to disciplinary action. Time and effort is necessary to promote the idea of the usefulness of clinical incident reporting before initiating such a system in an obstetric department. Staff need guidance as to which particular incidents to report (Table 6.1) and be encouraged to report by emphasising that the purpose of such a system is to provide opportunities for learning, identifying and rectifying mistakes, such that similar incidents will be less likely to occur. The purpose of incident reporting is not to discipline staff; the only exceptions to this would be criminal or malicious activities, acts of gross misconduct and repeated incidents.[4] When staff are converted to the idea that some good will come of their practice in reporting incidents, the floodgates may be opened! Inevitably, over-reporting of trivial incidents will occur, but should not be discouraged as this may adversely influence reporting of other, more serious events.

### MONITORING AND ANALYSIS OF INCIDENTS

There are two objectives in evaluating reported clinical incidents: (i) to investigate the individual characteristics of the case, including the involvement

**Table 6.1** Obstetric clinical incidents reported at Peterborough Hospitals NHS Trust

Drug errors and reactions
Failure to obtain consent
Near misses
Surgical/anaesthetic mishap
Untoward patient injury/death
Missed/delayed diagnosis
Complications following investigative or operative procedure
Incident potentially giving rise to a complaint or litigation
Any untoward outcome
Babies admitted unexpectedly to SCBU
Babies requiring intubation unexpectedly
Babies with Apgar below 6 at 5 min
Unexpected stillbirth
Shoulder dystocia
Hysterectomy
Bladder injury
Delay in obtaining urgently requested laboratory results influencing
        obstetric management
Faulty equipment

of health professionals; and (ii) to have a broader overview of all clinical incidents, looking at common recurring themes, identifying tasks prone to error, and appreciating many of the background factors surrounding a case.[5]

It must be recognised that incident reporting will never be universal – those lead obstetricians with responsibility for risk management must remain vigilant and seek out unreported cases through their day-to-day clinical work, and by conversation with their medical colleagues and those in midwifery management.[6]

A computerised maternity information system, where certain outcomes could be flagged up as qualifying for incident reporting, would greatly enhance comprehensive incident reporting. Reliable information technology can prove to be an extremely useful tool if it provides regular and accurate figures on the incidents of certain obstetric complications (e.g. failed instrumental delivery, postpartum haemorrhage, etc.). By constant monitoring of the incidence of these events, an insidious trend could be recognised early. Without a computerised maternity information system such figures are extremely difficult to come by and the task of collecting them is laborious and time consuming, as well as being of limited accuracy. Several specific benefits of such a system are listed in Table 6.2.

Some clinical incidents highlight a specific deficiency: in one obstetric unit a 'near miss' intrapartum stillbirth demonstrated that the skills of midwives in interpreting electronic fetal heart rate monitoring had lapsed seriously. This is one of several clinical incidents where it is possible to put in place remedial action which should improve the quality of clinical care.

## ANALYSIS OF THE HUMAN FACTORS

This area of risk management is an exciting field with the potential to produce a more fundamental change in the way we try to reduce the impact of human error. This approach involves looking at the human component within complex socio-technical systems. By looking at the type of incident that has occurred, it may be possible to identify a small number of doctors or other health professionals who are repeatedly prone to practices that deviate from accepted norms. In the absence of other confounding factors, such as stress and exhaustion (which are recognised to increase significantly the chance of error), their actions may be a consequence of their own inherent personality traits.[7] In such instances, sanctions and exhortations, re-training and the provision of new guidelines for procedures may not be helpful, but other approaches to enhance human performance may be necessary.[8] For a more detailed analysis of the human factors affecting clinical risk the reader is referred to the chapter by James Reason.[9]

## CHANGING BEHAVIOUR

Measures to change or influence behaviour of groups of professionals include audit, education and professional assessments performed as part of the Calman Training Programme. These assessments must include both verbal evidence directly from the trainee and practical evidence (from observation of

**Table 6.2** Impact of computerised pregnancy information on clinical risk

| Requirement | Problem | Example | Litigation risk | Financial cost | Expected benefit |
|---|---|---|---|---|---|
| Patient-based information should be legible | Handwriting may be illegible, signatures unreadable | May be unable to identify member of staff responsible for error | Likely effect | Legal claim | Readable entries, could automatically identify staff member |
| Patient-based information should be immediately available | Information contained in patient-held notes, hospital notes, PAS, laboratory systems, GP systems | Important details may be unknown (e.g. drug allergy, medical condition) or not available when patient is not present or forgets patient-held notes | Likely effect | Legal claim; inefficient use of resources | Optimise information availability and presentation (e.g. automatic prompts for side-effects, contra-indications, reduce duplication of investigations) |
| Patient-based information should be complete | Cannot ensure data capture in manual system | Additional procedure may not be recorded, details which may have a bearing on future pregnancies may not be captured (e.g. fetal head position at Caesarean section) | Likely effect | Possible loss of revenue from purchaser | Can make data items mandatory and prompt for additional procedures |
| Patient data should be proof against tampering | Patient-held records may be altered without being apparent | Patient altered date of delivery resulting in delivery of premature baby | Likely effect | Legal claim | Patient data would be robust and resistant to interference |
| Data required for audit | Manual system involves large effort, errors more likely, much audit not attempted because data items not readily available | Fetal abnormality database | Likely effect | Legal claim, possible cost-saving from targeting of resources to specific groups | Numerous useful audits could be undertaken to assess deviation from treatment protocols, outcome in sub-groups (e.g. high-risk pregnancies) |
| Clinical protocols should be adhered to | Staff may overlook or be unaware of protocol | Swabs not always taken from women with ruptured membranes, specific actions may not be performed in rare situations | Likely effect | Legal claim | System could provide automated prompts and monitor adherence to protocols. Risk management improved |

*Reproduced by kind permission from Mr M R Lumb.*

that individual) that a necessary skill has been attained or procedure is able to be performed.[10]

## IN PRACTICE

At Peterborough Hospitals NHS Trust, obstetric clinical incidents are reported on a simple form comprising one side of A4 in triplicate. Books of forms are located in all clinical areas. One copy is sent to the Obstetric Lead Clinician (SAS), one to the assistant general manager and the third to the Risk and Litigation Department. Dealing with the forms takes a significant amount of time, although many require no further action and are duly filed. An approximate and subjective grading system is used to classify incidents from the most serious (A) to relatively trivial (C). Many of the incidents reported provide an opportunity for discussion at clinical case review meetings and at regular weekly teaching sessions on cardiotograph (CTG) interpretation skills for midwives and doctors. Some cases require case-notes to be scrutinised and staff interviewed with a meticulous investigation of the events. A sensitive and non-threatening approach is required when staff are interviewed after clinical incidents. Such interviews provide an opportunity for education and constructive appraisal, to help both midwives and doctors in their professional development. Ideally, these are performed promptly as memories quickly fade. On rare occasions, a group of serious incidents with recurring themes involving the same individuals will require careful, prompt and drastic action to be taken by senior clinicians and management, if patient safety is thought to be at risk.

It may be appropriate to look at whether an incident has occurred through lack of clinical guidelines for that situation. However, a false sense of security may be engendered if such a 'quick fix' is not the most effective action to take but is **believed** to be so by those responsible for acting on incidents. Looking at the broader picture may be more appropriate. A monthly or quarterly report of clinical incidents, categorising them (e.g. equipment failure, communication breakdown, etc.) may provide a useful pointer as to the main problems. Considerable time is required to take both the detailed and broader look at all clinical incidents, and this is often beyond the capabilities of the consultant obstetrician, unless a dedicated session is allocated for this work.

Serious incidents will often require that statements are written by midwifery and medical staff concerning their involvement in the case. Guidance and support are necessary as staff often find this task stressful and worrying. At Peterborough Hospitals NHS Trust, we provide written guidelines and personal supervision to our medical trainees in writing such statements.

## ERRORS AND 'NEAR MISSES'

Errors and near misses will inevitably occur and should be seen positively as an opportunity for learning and professional development. We all learn from our mistakes, and indeed 'near misses' can serve to modify an individual's practice by the occasional experience of such errors. These, therefore, can been seen as serving to maintain the proper level of skill. Most medical trainees, having 'crossed the boundary', will find the experience a salutary one and will be less likely to follow the same course of action in their future practice.[11]

## INTRAPARTUM CARE

The appropriate management of intrapartum care is the time of greatest risk in the management of a pregnant woman. The organisation of medical staff responsible for the labour ward has evolved over the last few years, with the recognition of the importance of dedicated consultant obstetrician sessions. All Trusts should now be working towards the recommendations of the Joint RCOG/RCM Working Party on Organisational Standards for delivery suites to provide at least 10 fixed consultant labour ward sessions throughout the working week.[12] This argument is logically progressed to a situation where a consultant is available 24 hours a day, 7 days a week, but the personal, political and financial implications of such a proposal are considerable. The immediate availability of a consultant obstetrician is even more crucial given the impact of Calman training on the experience of medical trainees, the reduction in trainees' working hours and the tendency for the senior house officer grade to be more an observational role than one involving a significant service input. The consultant often finds himself or herself, therefore, performing somewhat routine tasks that were previously performed at registrar or even SHO level. Maternity units also have a duty to achieve a realistic midwifery establishment to enhance safety by providing an appropriate midwife to patient ratio.[12]

### ELECTRONIC FETAL HEART RATE MONITORING (EFHRM)

Deficiencies in interpretation of cardiotocographs (CTGs) were identified as being a significant factor by the Confidential Enquiry into Stillbirths and Deaths in Infancy.[13] At Peterborough Hospitals NHS Trust, significant time and effort has been invested in establishing a regular weekly educational session for midwives and medical trainees, looking specifically at CTG interpretation skills. These educational sessions begin with tutorials on fetal physiology and acid-base regulation in a fetus, and move on to group discussions and reviews of specific cases. This practice has enhanced the general level of knowledge of interpretation of CTGs and has increased the professionalism involved in discussing this particular form of monitoring. Both medical and midwifery staff can lapse into sloppy terminology when describing CTGs: 'it looks a bit flat' or 'I think the baby is a bit sleepy' or 'the FH is dipping a bit'. The general use of consistent terminology has improved and has assisted the discussion between medical trainees and consultants, supported also by fax links between consultants' homes and the labour ward. As a result of the weekly CTG teaching sessions, a significant educational resource has been built up of prime examples of CTG abnormalities. This is akin to the collection termed the 'Crimson File',[12] which is an additional useful educational resource well worth acquiring and using. At Peterborough Hospitals NHS Trust, we have introduced the 'Crimson

# CTG Learning points No. 1

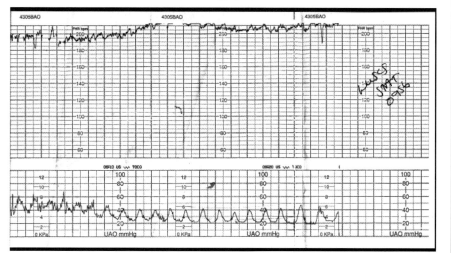

# Frequent low-amplitude contractions are strongly suggestive of
# PLACENTAL ABRUPTION

**Fig. 6.1** CTG learning points

File' to medical trainees at the start of their appointment. Computer software programmes are available that provide training in CTG interpretation and are simple to use. All new medical trainees should be encouraged to work through such programmes at an early stage of their training, and midwives likewise. Records may be kept of which individuals have actually progressed through the programmes, thereby monitoring uptake.

## 'LEARNING POINTS'

The best examples of CTG abnormalities with a single written 'learning point' added can be laminated and placed at strategic points throughout the maternity unit. If these are in eye-catching colours, staff having coffee cannot help but notice them on the bulletin board and hopefully recognise the pattern and remember the message if they encounter it at a later date (Fig. 6.1).

## FORCEPS/VENTOUSE DELIVERY

Instrumental delivery is a potential source of complaints and litigation. Litigation cases associated with the death of a baby are often characterised by both inadequate fetal heart rate monitoring or mismanagement of forceps delivery, as well as poor supervision by senior staff.[14] Consultant obstetricians must recognise that the levels of competency in such obstetric skills of current Calman trainees may be significantly less than those expected of the traditional senior registrars. Greater supervision and education is, therefore, needed, and instrumental delivery should ideally be audited regularly, looking particularly at 'failed trials' of instrumental delivery. The general inclination to use the Ventouse as the instrument of choice (still the subject of debate)[15] has led to an attitude by medical trainees that the accurate determination of fetal head position is no longer important. At Peterborough Hospitals NHS Trust, detailed and precise guidelines for instrumental delivery were included in our labour ward guidelines after a number of clinical incidents, and the recognition of a rising trend in failed instrumental deliveries.

## CAESAREAN SECTION

All units are likely to be experiencing a significant rise in the rate of Caesarean section, the reasons for which are beyond the scope of this chapter. A useful educational intervention we have adopted at Peterborough Hospitals NHS Trust is to include a regular Caesarean section case review for the first hour of our weekly postgraduate teaching session, critically appraising the clinical management of specific cases.

## 'PRACTICE RUNS'

Variously referred to as 'practice runs', 'dry runs' or 'fire drills', the practice of rehearsing a response to a particular clinical problem such as shoulder dystocia is thought to enhance performance when that situation arises in reality. Various models are available to practise obstetric and midwifery skills, for example in shoulder dystocia. This particular area could be further developed with computer simulations of clinical situations which test responses.

## CLINICAL GUIDELINES

Clinical guidelines can be defined as 'systematically developed statements designed to help practitioners and patients make decisions about appropriate healthcare for specific circumstances'.[16] The effect of clinical guidelines should be to reduce inappropriate variations in practice. They should provide valuable guidance in specific clinical situations and thereby promote good practice. Practice may be described as 'following' a guideline or 'deviating' from a guideline. The term 'violation of a guideline' is less desirable and may be confused with the term 'violation' used to define a certain type of clinical error.[9] The application of clinical guidelines involves several key stages which, in turn, will influence the effectiveness of the guidelines in practice.

## METHODOLOGY OF DEVELOPMENT

Guidelines should be based wherever possible on sound scientific evidence. The National Institute of Clinical Excellence (NICE) will be responsible for the development of guidelines.[17] Currently, guidelines may be derived from various sources including, for example consensus statements and 'expert' panels; however, such groups of individuals may have incomplete knowledge of all the published work on that topic. The role of NICE is to ensure that the best evidence-based medicine is the basis on which guidelines will be produced.[18] The Royal College of Obstetricians and Gynaecologists is to set up a Clinical Effectiveness and Standards Board (CESB) which will also be responsible for producing a co-ordinated and structured programme of guidelines.[19] The RCOG has already produced the 'green top' series of guidelines under the direction of the Scientific Advisory Committee which, to date, includes 10 guidelines relating to obstetrical topics. Locally produced guidelines must be drawn up with involvement from those professionals at the 'sharp end' of clinical practice with representation from midwives, medical trainees, consultant obstetricians and other health professionals where appropriate. Guidelines must be readily accessible and easy to follow if they are to be effective.

## IMPLEMENTATION

Effective implementation of clinical guidelines is not achieved by passive dissemination. Active steps are essential to educate staff about the guidelines, the basis on which they have been formulated, the purpose for which they have been derived, and the clinical steps involved in putting them into practice, particularly if new guidelines differ significantly from previous practice. There is evidence that properly developed guidelines can change clinical practice and are, therefore, likely to lead to changes in patient outcome.[20–22] Many units produce sound, workable guidelines but are thwarted by a failure of staff to comply with them. Why should this be so? What are the barriers to successful implementation and what enhances adherence to clinical guidelines?. The evidence suggests that a variety of strategies are necessary to highlight the good practice described in clinical guidelines and that educational interventions seem to have the best effect.[23] Tackling the problem from several different angles may prove to be most effective, an approach which is also likely to help in other areas of maintaining standards, such as record-keeping (see below). For example, not only perform a clinical audit of adherence to a certain guideline, but refer to guidelines, where appropriate, during regular case review meetings, ward rounds, perinatal mortality meetings, etc., or whenever the opportunity arises.[24] Currently, evidence is insufficient to reach firm conclusions about the relative effectiveness of different educational and implementation strategies in relation to clinical guidelines and research is ongoing. The RCOG has initiated work in collaboration with the National Centre for Clinical Audit (NCCA) on the uptake and use of guidelines.[25]

## CONFIDENTIAL ENQUIRIES

The Confidential Enquiry into Stillbirths and Deaths in Infancy (CESDI) and the Confidential Enquiry into Maternal Deaths (CEMD) are valuable sources of evidence of deficiencies in clinical practice defined as substandard care.

**Table 6.3** The Peterborough Hospitals NHS Trust checklist of the topics for discussion when counselling a woman regarding amniocentesis

TO BE FILED IN HOSPITAL NOTES

Patient's label                    Date _____

AMNIOCENTESIS

Checklist for staff

Tick box

Procedure explained - - - - - - - - - - - - - - - - - - - - - - - - - - - - - - - - - - - - - - - -

Risk of miscarriage is 1 in 200 - - - - - - - - - - - - - - - - - - - - - - - - - - - - - -

Results available after 2–3 weeks - - - - - - - - - - - - - - - - - - - - - - - - -

Risk of culture failure is 0.5% - - - - - - - - - - - - - - - - - - - - - - - - - - - -

Amniocentesis will detect only major chromosomal
re-arrangements and not all minor deletions - - - - - - - - - - - - - - - -

Method of termination explained if chosen after abnormal results

Explained by          - - - - - - - - - - - - - - - - - - - - - - - - - - - - - - - - - - - - - - PRINT NAME

Signature:          - - - - - - - - - - - - - - - - - - - - - - - - - - - - - - - - - - - - - -

Status:          SENIOR SHO / REGISTRAR / STAFF GRADE
                 SENIOR REGISTRAR / CONSULTANT

Following publication of such enquiries, each maternity unit should form a small group of professionals, including both midwives and doctors, to examine the recommendations and produce a brief 'action plan' for the early implementation of those recommendations. Such enquiries are accepted as a respected source of advice in the legal context, and generally assumed to be followed, unless there are compelling local reasons not to do so.

## CHECKLISTS

Structured documentation or proformas, either on paper or computer, may provide the opportunity for greater adherence to guidelines.[26] At Peterborough Hospitals NHS Trust, we have developed checklists for a variety of clinical situations such as: the assessment of risk of thrombo-embolism prior to emergency or planned Caesarean section, the topics for discussion when counselling a woman regarding amniocentesis (Table 6.3), and a comprehensive checklist with tick boxes of all the issues involved in maternal serum screening pre-test counselling.

## MAINTENANCE OF GUIDELINES

Guidelines should be dated and referenced, with small amendments being necessary on a regular basis, as evidence and information becomes available from various sources. Any changes to guidelines should be dated. It is important to retain former versions of guidelines as they may be required for reference in future complaints or litigation where the standard will be judged against the guidelines for practice that existed at that time. Every 2 years or so, a major overhaul of the guidelines is usually necessary.

## CLINICAL NEGLIGENCE SCHEME FOR TRUSTS (CNST)

The CNST produces a list of obstetric standards and specific topics which require to be covered by clinical guidelines.[19]

## RECORD-KEEPING STANDARDS

Record-keeping standards vary enormously between individuals. In general, medical staff tend to have lower standards of record-keeping than midwives. Failures of care are often attributable to poor communication and, therefore, there must be a strong philosophy within a maternity unit that high standards of record-keeping are desirable and worth attaining.[27] A significant amount of effort is required, however, to demonstrate both this philosophy and to measure the extent to which standards are maintained. Record-keeping standards are readily auditable. Such an audit can be undertaken in a variety of ways. At Peterborough Hospitals NHS Trust, a hospital-wide record-keeping audit is undertaken by our Clinical Audit Department on a regular basis as part of the requirement for CNST accreditation. At a more local level, our Practice Development Midwife encourages the involvement of both midwives and medical trainees in record-keeping audits, looking at adherence to a number of different standards (e.g. name signed and printed underneath with designation on the first entry, vaginal examinations entered in red ink, each new page of notes carries the patient's name and hospital number with the date at the top of the left hand margin, etc.). It is important that medical trainees as well as midwives are involved in this exercise since those two groups are the professionals who contribute most in volume to the patient's records. An exercise involving self-audit, where the individual assesses their own record keeping standards as part of the midwifery supervisory system, may result in a more critical assessment and bring home to that individual the areas needing improvement. A similar exercise could be undertaken with medical trainees as part of their Calman assessments. Again, a multi-faceted approach to this area may result in improved standards. At Peterborough Hospitals NHS Trust, we take any opportunity to assess record keeping standards, for example at our regular clinical case reviews, such as the weekly Caesarean section case review, perinatal mortality meetings, ward rounds, etc. Highlighting the importance of this issue repeatedly helps to bring the message home, so long as the approach is informal, non-threatening and non-judgmental. Certain specific guidelines on record-keeping will be likely to have a direct impact on clinical care and facilitate good communication between professionals. As a specific example of how a guideline can improve care, I will quote a case of a pregnant woman admitted to a maternity unit on many occasions with unexplained abdominal pain throughout her pregnancy. A retrospective diagnosis of a placental abruption was made after an emergency Caesarean section for fetal bradycardia. The patient reported afterwards that she did not feel that her symptoms were being taken seriously. At no point was a consultant obstetrician consulted about her antenatal management. On each occasion that she was admitted, the medical trainee documented the fact that she had 'several previous admissions' with a similar complaint. What was not evident, however, was that she had **15** previous admissions as no-one had taken the trouble to count them. We now follow a guideline which states that on completion of an antenatal admission entry into the case notes, a line is drawn across the page and the next admission numbered. After three admissions it is recommended that a consultant obstetrician is informed (if not already aware), to facilitate review by an experienced obstetrician.

The importance of high standards of record-keeping are emphasised on our induction day for new medical trainees. Dr Nicholas Norwell from the Medical Defence Union has published a humorous article (*Ten Commandments of Record-Keeping*) which can be a valuable resource at such induction days.[28] Consultants, perhaps, are often the worst offenders with regard to legibility of entries into notes and should, therefore, take note that we have a duty to show by example.

## EDUCATION AND AUDIT

The acquisition of factual knowledge and scientific evidence is obviously a vital part of risk management. Each maternity unit should strive to obtain for its midwives and doctors easy access to relevant medical and midwifery journals, the Internet, the Cochrane database and other important sources of information. At Peterborough Hospitals NHS Trust, we hold a regular weekly combined obstetric and paediatric meeting with a rolling programme of journal article review, perinatal morbidity, mortality and discussion of ongoing antenatal problems, as well as feedback from the Special Care Baby Unit. A regular postgraduate teaching afternoon plays an important role in general education with risk management covered as a specific topic.

## COMPLAINTS AND LITIGATION

Complaints are, not surprisingly, generally viewed negatively by doctors. They are seen as enormously time-consuming, often unjustified and frequently the source of considerable personal stress. The risk management policies outlined above will go some way to reducing the incidence of complaints. The positive side of complaints, however, is that they may highlight an area of deficiency hitherto unidentified; the patient involved often sees resolution of the complaint when they can see the changes made as a result of their actions. The postnatal period is a time when dissatisfaction may set in, as the perception by health professionals is one of reduced risk once the baby has been delivered. Staff allocation to postnatal wards is often seen as one of the lower priorities and medical trainees may not appreciate the value of returning to talk to a woman they have delivered to run through the labour and delivery, and explain the management. By encouraging such 'de-briefing', many women will have the opportunity to appreciate and understand fully what happened to them. This should not only enhance their long-term psychological health, but also reduce the likelihood of complaints and/or litigation.

## OBSTETRIC RISK MANAGEMENT GROUP

Various models exist across the UK of groups of health professionals set up to manage obstetric risk and to deal effectively with clinical incidents. At Peterborough Hospitals NHS Trust, we believe in keeping such a group small, as this appears to enhance its effectiveness. The group has been in existence for more than three years and comprises 2 consultant obstetricians, an obstetric anaesthetist, a practice development midwife, and 3 midwife managers. An agenda and minutes are produced and the group meets monthly. The agenda is often broad, ranging from discussions concerning an intermittent fault of the pH analyser on the labour ward, to the organisation of our Caesarean section lists, to discussion of recent serious clinical incidents. The minutes are circulated widely to our assistant general manager, midwifery managers, risk and litigation manager, and all clinical areas. Staff value and benefit from feedback regarding cases and this, in turn, helps to re-inforce acceptance of incident reporting.

### MEDICAL TRAINEES

The responsibility for supervision and education of medical trainees in a specialty that features so highly in clinical risk is an enormous one. The task could be achieved very much better if the consultant grade were significantly expanded. In my relatively short experience in clinical risk management, a number of common problems and themes can be identified amongst medical trainees' behaviour and clinical practice; some of these are very specific and some are more general. Specifically, a failure to refer to patient details by examining the wrist band has the potential for serious complications if blood transfusion is required. In general, a lack of attention to **detail** can have serious repercussions. Mistaking a histology report for a recent one rather than from the previous year could mislead the doctor into thinking that an ectopic pregnancy is highly unlikely – simple inattention to the date on this pathology report could lead to a failure to diagnose an ectopic pregnancy with serious consequences for the patient. Failure to examine in detail the antenatal notes of a patient may mean that a variety of risk factors are not taken into account during that woman's intrapartum care. Trainees should all be encouraged to refer to their patient by **name** and always refer to their name when discussing their management with the consultant. Without such an identifier the scope for misunderstanding, misinformation and mismanagement is enormous. The de-personalising of clinical care with comments such as 'room 3 is fully dilated' should be strongly discouraged.

## FAILURE OF DOCUMENTATION

All medical trainees should be encouraged to enter into the notes any conversations or discussions between themselves and the patient, and with their consultant. Whenever they are called to assess a woman in labour or comment upon a CTG, an entry should be made into the notes. It is not sufficient, and is inappropriate, to rely on the midwife to enter such an event into the records – it is the responsibility of the doctor concerned.

## CONCLUSIONS

Risk management in obstetrical practice represents an enormous challenge for the profession. Changes and improvements in practice may have profound

## Key points for clinical practice

- Risk management is about enhancing the safety of clinical care.

- Reporting and analysis of clinical incidents is vital.

- Staff are encouraged to report and learn from incidents.

- An Obstetric Risk Management Group will consider all areas of clinical risk and take effective action.

- Comprehensive clinical guidelines provide a framework for safe, effective management.

- Close supervision of intrapartum care by experienced obstetricians should occur at all times.

- A continuing programme of CTG interpretation will pay dividends.

- An intimate and accurate picture of a maternity unit's workload and practices can only be achieved through computerisation of maternity data.

- High standards should be set for record-keeping and strenuous efforts for constant improvement.

- Remember to praise when a job is well done!

and life-enhancing effects for our patients, both mother and baby. The pursuit of highest possible standards does require sufficient time, motivation and leadership as well as the appropriate information technology to provide data for audit, planning and monitoring of activities. This chapter has referred to simple and achievable strategies that help to reduce obstetric risk and enhance the safety of clinical practice.

## References

1 Vincent C. (ed) Clinical Risk Management, 2nd edn. London: BMJ Publishing Group, 1999; xv
2 Rigge M. Patient expectations of clinical governance. In: Lugon M, Secker-Walker J (eds) Clinical Governance – Making it happen, 1st edn. London: RSM, 1999; 6
3 Royal College of Obstetricians and Gynaecologists. Clinical Audit Unit, 9th Bulletin. London: RCOG, 1999
4 Secker-Walker J. Clinical risk management. In: Vincent C. (ed) Clinical Risk Management, 2nd edn. London: BMJ Publishing Group, 1999; 77–91
5 Stanhope N, Vincent C, Taylor-Adams SE, O'Connor AM, Beard RW. Applying human factors methods to clinical risk management in obstetrics. Br J Obstet Gynaecol 1997; 104: 1225–1232
6 Stanhope N, Crowley-Murphy M, Vincent C, O'Connor AM, Taylor-Adams SE. An evaluation of adverse incident reporting. J Eval Clin Pract 1999; 5: 5–12
7 Firth-Cozens J. Stress, psychological problems and clinical performance. In: Vincent C, Ennis M, Audley RJ. (eds) Medical Accidents. New York: Oxford University, 1993; 131–149
8 Cook RI, Woods DD. Operating at the sharp end: the complexity of human error. In: Bogner MS. (ed) Human Errors in Medicine. Hillsdale, NJ: Erlbaum, 1994: 255–310
9 Reason J. Understanding adverse events: human factors. In: Vincent C. (ed) Clinical Risk Management, 2nd edn. London: BMJ Publishing Group, 1999; 31–54
10 Firth-Cozens J. Tackling risk by changing behaviour. In: Vincent C. (ed) Clinical Risk Management, 2nd edn. London: BMJ Publishing Group, 1999; 55–72
11 Rasmussen J. Human error and the problem of causality in analysis of accidents. Philos Trans R Soc Lond Biol Sci 1990; 327: 449–462
12 Royal College of Obstetricians and Gynaecologists. Towards Safer Childbirth. London: RCOG, 1999
13 Confidential Enquiry into Stillbirths and Deaths in Infancy. 4th Annual Report. London: CESDI, 1997;
14 Ennis M, Vincent C. Obstetric accidents: a review of 64 cases. BMJ 1990; 300: 1365–1367
15 Royal College of Obstetricians and Gynaecologists. Debate at RCOG meeting: Modern Management of Labour, Liverpool, April 1999
16 Field MJ, Lohr KN. (eds) Guidelines for Clinical Practice from Development to Use. Washington, DC: National Academy, 1992
17 Department of Health. A First Class Service: Quality in the New NHS. London: Department of Health, 1998
18 Jackson R, Feder G. Guidelines for clinical guidelines. BMJ 1998; 317: 427–428
19 Royal College of Obstetricians and Gynaecologists. Maintaining Good Medical Practice in Obstetrics and Gynaecology. London: RCOG, 1999
20 Anon. Implementing Clinical Practice Guidelines: can guidelines be used to improve clinical practice?. Effective Health Care, Bulletin No. 8. University of Leeds, 1994
21 Grimshaw JM, Russell IT. Effect of clinical guidelines on medical practice: a systematic review of rigorous evaluations. Lancet 1993; 342: 1317–1322
22 Thomas LH, McColl E, Cullum N, Rousseau N, Soutter J, Steen N. Effect of clinical guidelines in nursing, midwifery and the therapies: a systematic review of evaluations. Qual Health Care 1998; 7: 183–191
23 Grimshaw J, Freemantle N, Wallace S et al. Developing and implementing clinical practice guidelines. Qual Health Care 1995; 4: 55–64

24 Wensing M, Grol R. Single and combined strategies for implementing changes in primary care: a literature review. Int J Qual Health Care 1994; 6: 115–132

25 Royal College of Obstetricians and Gynaecologists. Clinical Governance: Setting Standards to Improve Women's Health. London: RCOG, 1999

26 Lilford RJ, Kelly M, Baines A et al. Effect of using protocols on medical care: randomised trial of three methods of taking an antenatal history. BMJ 1992; 305: 1181–1184

27. Confidential Enquiry into Stillbirths and Deaths in Infancy. 6th Annual Report. London: CESDI, 1999

28 Norwell N. The ten commandments of record-keeping. J Med Defence Union 1997; 13: 1

*Alastair MacLennan for the*
*International Cerebral Palsy Task Force*

# A template for defining a causal relationship between acute intrapartum events and cerebral palsy

## AN INTERNATIONAL CONSENSUS STATEMENT

This debate was initiated by the Perinatal Society of Australia and New Zealand and the Consensus Statement has been supported by the following colleges and scientific societies.

*American College of Obstetricians and Gynecologists*
*American Gynecological and Obstetrical Society*
*Australian College of Midwives*
*Hong Kong College of Obstetricians and Gynaecologists*
*Hong Kong Society of Neonatal Medicine*
*Institute of Obstetrics and Gynaecology of The Royal College of Physicians of Ireland*
*International Society of Perinatal Obstetricians*
*New Zealand College of Midwives*
*Paediatric Society of New Zealand*
*Royal Australasian College of Physicians, Paediatric Division*
*Royal Australian College of General Practitioners*
*Royal Australian College of Obstetricians and Gynaecologists*
*Royal College of Obstetricians & Gynaecologists*
*Royal College of Pathologists of Australasia*
*Royal New Zealand College of Obstetricians & Gynaecologists*
*Society of Obstetricians and Gynaecologists of Canada*

## CHAIRMAN'S FOREWORD

In 1997, the research committee of the Perinatal Society of Australia and New Zealand competitively funded a special initiative to bring together the modern literature on the causation of cerebral palsy, and to try to define an objective

**Prof. Alastair MacLennan** (Chairperson), Department of Obstetrics and Gynaecology, University of Adelaide, Women's & Children's Hospital, 72 King William Road, North Adelaide, SA 5006, Australia.
alastair.maclennan@medicine.adelaide.edu.au

template of evidence to better identify cases of cerebral palsy where the neuropathology began or became established around labour and birth. There have recently been many advances in a wide variety of scientific areas associated with cerebral palsy and thus this multidisciplinary review may benefit research into the causation and prevention of cerebral palsy and may also help those who offer expert opinion when counselling in this area or give such opinion in court.

The corresponding task force was open to anyone who could make a scientific contribution to understanding in this area. The task force had representation from a wide range of clinical and scientific specialties. Submissions were sought from the society's 1000 membership which includes scientists, pathologists, obstetricians, neonatalogists, midwives, neonatal nurses and epidemiologists. International contributions were sought from those identified from the current literature as contributing to this area through peer reviewed research. They were not pre-selected for their views and they were invited to join the corresponding task force. Some international members joined later in the discussion process as word of this open debate reached them.

During 1997 and 1998, multiple on-line electronic conferences were held and in March 1998 many of the task force members were able to participate in a workshop in Alice Springs, Australia to discuss the fourth draft of the statement. Drafts of the statement were circulated and debated with the sixth draft being discussed at an international telephone conference in October 1998. The paper continued to be redrafted eight times until consensus was reached. No opinion was excluded from the debate but the statement only includes discussion that has a reasonable scientific basis and can be referenced. All members agree that updated reports will be required within a few years when further information is published. It is hoped that other international researchers in this area will offer to assist in future statements. The final draft of the statement was sent to the professional colleges and scientific societies to which the task force members belong. To date, no such group has declined to support the statement or has disputed its final content. A list of professional bodies endorsing the statement at the time of publication is included in the consensus statement.

Consensus was reached with some difficulty in two areas. The first was the current validity of neuro-imaging in the infant or child to retrospectively determine the precise perinatal timing, pathology or cause of the abnormalities seen on imaging. The task force awaits the publication of strong data, using the criteria suggested in its template, to define an acute intrapartum hypoxic event to validate specific neuro-imaging appearances that occur as a result of acute intrapartum hypoxia. These images must be different from those which arise following chronic asphyxial or non-asphyxial causes of cerebral palsy in order to be of help in determining intrapartum timing.

The second area of debate was terminology and in particular the term 'non-reassuring fetal status' was debated. It has been adopted in the consensus statement rather than the term 'fetal distress' as clinical signs often poorly predict a compromised fetus and continued use of this latter term may encourage wrong assumptions or inappropriate management.

The task force acknowledges that some cases of cerebral palsy probably originate in labour. By defining these cases it should also help focus research on the many antenatal causes of cerebral palsy and their prevention as well as the prevention of intrapartum asphyxia which has been the major clinical goal to date. I thank all those who have donated their time, expertise and support to the compilation of this consensus statement.

## INTERNATIONAL CEREBRAL PALSY TASK FORCE MEMBERS

### Chairperson:

*Associate Professor Alastair MacLennan, (Obstetrician), Department of Obstetrics and Gynaecology, University of Adelaide, Women's & Children's Hospital, 72 King William Road, North Adelaide, SA 5006, Australia*
*Tel: +61 8 8204 7619; Fax: +61 8 8204 7652*
*E-mail: amaclennan@medicine.adelaide.edu.au*

Dr Nadia Badawi, (Neonatologist), The New Children's Hospital, New South Wales, Australia

Dr Laura Bennet, (Fetal Physiologist), The University of Auckland, New Zealand

Prof. Michael Bennett, (Obstetrician), University of New South Wales, Australia

Dr Eve Blair, (Epidemiologist), Institute of Child Health Research, Western Australia, Australia

Prof. John Bonnar, (Obstetrician), Trinity College, Ireland

Prof. Max Brinsmead, (Obstetrician), John Hunter Hospital, New South Wales, Australia

Dr Helen Chambers, (Pathologist), King Edward Memorial & Princess Margaret Hospitals, Western Australia, Australia

Prof. Paul Colditz, (Neonatologist), University of Queensland, Australia

Dr Robert Creasy, (Obstetrician), University of Texas, USA

Assoc. Prof. Brian Darlow, (Paediatrician), University

of Otago, Christchurch, New Zealand

Dr John Doig, (Obstetrician), University of Otago, Christchurch, New Zealand

Ms Kerena Eckert, (Research Midwife), University of Adelaide, South Australia, Australia

Prof. David Edwards, (Neonatologist), University of London, UK

Dr Margaret Furness, (Radiologist), Women's & Children's Hospital, South Australia, Australia

Dr Alistair Jan Gunn, (Paediatrician), The University of Auckland, New Zealand

Dr Eric Haan, (Clinical Geneticist), Women's & Children's Hospital, South Australia, Australia

Dr Tina Hayward, (Radiologist), Women's & Children's Hospital, South Australia, Australia

Dr Sue Jacobs, (Obstetrician), King George V Hospital, New South Wales, Australia

Dr Ann Johnson, (Epidemiologist), National

Perinatal Epidemiology Unit, Oxford, UK

Dr John Keogh, (Obstetrician), Hornsby Ku-Ring-Gai Hospital, New South Wales, Australia

Prof. Marc Keirse, (Obstetrician), Flinders University, South Australia, Australia

Dr James King, (Obstetrician), The Mater Perinatal Epidemiology Unit, Queensland, Australia

Prof. Robert Lea, (Obstetrician), University of Halifax, Canada

Dr James Low, (Obstetrician), Queen's University, Canada

Dr Ian McKenzie, (Obstetrician), University of Oxford, UK

Dr Andrew McPhee, (Neonatologist), Women's & Children's Hospital, South Australia, Australia

Prof. Yuji Murata, (Obstetrician), Osaka University, Japan

Prof. John Newnham, (Obstetrician), King Edward Memorial Hospital, Western Australia, Australia

Dr John O'Loughlin,
(Obstetrician), Past
President, Royal Australian
College of Obstetricians &
Gynaecologists, Australia

Dr Robert Ouvrier,
(Paediatric Neurologist),
New Children's Hospital,
New South Wales, Australia

Prof. Bill Parer,
(Obstetrician), University of
California, San Francisco,
USA

Prof. Jeffrey Perlman,
(Neonatologist), University
of Texas, Dallas, USA

Dr Sandra Rees,
(Neuroscientist), The
University of Melbourne,
Victoria, Australia

Dr Rosemary Reid,
(Obstetrician), University of
Otago, Christchurch, New
Zealand

Prof. Robert Resnik,
(Obstetrician), University of
California, San Diego, USA

Assoc. Prof. Greg Rice,
(Perinatal Scientist),
Univeristy of Melbourne,
Victoria, Australia

Prof. Knox Ritchie,
(Obstetrician), University of
Toronto, Canada

Dr Roberto Romero,
(Obstetrician), Wayne State
University, Detroit, USA

Prof. Jeffrey Robinson,
(Obstetrician), The
University of Adelaide,
South Australia, Australia

Mr John Spencer,
(Obstetrician), Northwick
Park Hospital, UK

Prof. Fiona Stanley,
(Epidemiologist), Institute
of Child Health Research,
Western Australia, Australia

Dr Leon Stern,
(Rehabilitation Physician),
Women's & Children's
Hospital, South Australia,
Australia

Dr Peter Stone,
(Obstetrician), University of
Auckland, New Zealand

Dr John Svigos,
(Obstetrician), Women's &
Children's Hospital, South
Australia, Australia

Prof Malcolm Symonds,
(Obstetrician), University of
Nottingham, UK

Dr Jenny Westgate,
(Obstetrician), University of
Auckland, New Zealand

Dr Andrea Witlin,
(Obstetrician), University of
Texas, Galveston, USA

Prof. Victor Yu,
(Neonatologist), Monash
University, Victoria,
Australia

## INTRODUCTION

New insights into the origins of cerebral palsy have recently transformed the old concept that most cases of cerebral palsy begin in labour. There are many causes including developmental abnormalities,[1,2] metabolic abnormalities,[3] autoimmune and coagulation disorders[4] and infections[5] in addition to trauma and hypoxia (asphyxia)[6,7] in the fetus and newborn. Efforts to identify possible causes of cerebral palsy require skills from many disciplines.

Contrary to previous beliefs and assumptions, clinical epidemiological studies indicate that, in the majority of cases, the events leading to cerebral palsy occur in the fetus prior to the onset of labour or in the newborn following delivery.[8,9] However, in a given clinical scenario, it is difficult to assess which features indicate causes contributing to the adverse outcome. This is particularly true before delivery, when the clinical measures used for the assessment of fetal well-being are almost always indirect and generally inadequate to assess fetal brain function.

The problem for the individual case is that it is very difficult to identify, retrospectively, antenatal causes of cerebral palsy. Conversely, damaging hypoxia (asphyxia) during labour can be suspected from many clinical signs, none of which are specific to damaging hypoxia and which could, therefore, reflect other conditions in the fetus.[10] By combining some of these clinical signs with certain objective investigations, hypoxia during labour may be more reliably ascertained. The timing of the onset of hypoxia, i.e. antenatal or intrapartum, requires further evidence that is discussed in this statement.

## TERMINOLOGY

This Task Force re-iterates a previous consensus statement,[11] that the terms 'fetal distress' and 'birth asphyxia' are inappropriate and should not be used clinically. This opinion is endorsed by the American College of Obstetricians and Gynecologists[12] and the Society of Obstetricians and Gynaecologists of Canada.[13] The term 'fetal distress' should be replaced by the term 'non-reassuring fetal status' and a description of the clinical sign or test in question that led to that conclusion, e.g. pathological fetal acidaemia as defined by an umbilical arterial cord pH < 7.0.

The term 'asphyxia' is defined experimentally as impaired respiratory gas exchange accompanied by the development of metabolic acidosis. It is usually reserved for experimental situations when these changes can be accurately established. In the clinical context, 'fetal asphyxia' is progressive hypoxaemia and hypercapnia with a significant metabolic acidaemia.[14,15] In practice, the timing of the onset and the progression of these changes can be difficult or impossible to ascertain. When possible, the timing of factors should be described as 'fetal' or 'antenatal' if they occur before the onset of labour; as 'intrapartum' if they occur or recur between onset of labour and complete expulsion of the baby and 'neonatal' if they occur after the birth has been completed. 'Perinatal asphyxia' can be used when the timing is uncertain. Factors may also be described as 'acute' (occurring within a brief time period such as hours) or 'chronic' (in which case they may commence in one period and continue into subsequent periods over days or weeks) and as 'continuous' or 'intermittent'.

'Neonatal encephalopathy' is a clinically defined syndrome of disturbed neurological function in the term or near-term infant during the first week after birth, manifested by difficulty with initiating and maintaining respiration, depression of tone and reflexes, altered level of consciousness and often by seizures.[16] It is less clear which clinical signs indicate disturbed neurological function in very preterm infants. We have chosen not to use the diagnosis 'hypoxic ischaemic encephalopathy' in this template as hypoxia and ischaemia have often not been proved and have been assumed from a variety of clinical markers that do not accurately reflect hypoxia and ischaemia of either acute or chronic origin.[16] Over 75% of cases of neonatal encephalopathy have no clinical signs of intrapartum hypoxia.[17–20]

## PROBLEMS IN DEFINING THE CAUSE AND TIMING OF THE NEUROPATHOLOGY CAUSING CEREBRAL PALSY

Cerebral palsy, which is characterised by non-progressive, abnormal control of movement or posture, is not diagnosed until months or years after birth. Retrospective review of the pregnancy records often cannot reveal any obvious antenatal cause because fetal brain development and function cannot currently be routinely visualised or monitored.

## COMPLICATIONS OCCURRING IN THE ANTEPARTUM PERIOD ARE COMMON AND IMPORTANT CAUSES OF CEREBRAL PALSY

Epidemiological studies suggest that, in about 90% of cases, intrapartum hypoxia could not be the cause of cerebral palsy and that, in the remaining 10%, intrapartum signs compatible with damaging hypoxia may have had antenatal or intrapartum origins.[21,22] These studies demonstrate that a large proportion of cases are associated with maternal and antenatal factors such as prematurity, intra-uterine growth restriction, intra-uterine infection, fetal coagulation disorders, multiple pregnancy, antepartum haemorrhage, breech presentation, chromosomal or congenital anomalies.[1–11,23–25]

Signs of fetal compromise, such as changes in fetal heart rate and passage of meconium, are neither sensitive nor specific to any particular cause and only sometimes indicate damaging intrapartum hypoxia.[26] When metabolic acidaemia has been conclusively proven by fetal, umbilical and/or very early neonatal blood gases, it remains to be proven whether this is attributable to a chronic or intermittent hypoxia of long-standing duration (e.g. days and weeks) or whether a *de novo* acute hypoxia has occurred during labour or birth in a previously healthy fetus. Intra-uterine growth restriction may sometimes be associated with chronic hypoxia and cerebral palsy.[27] Animal studies show that induced, prolonged placental insufficiency in the last third of gestation resulting in persistent moderate fetal hypoxaemia disrupts myelination and the growth of the cerebellum.[28] They also demonstrate that, in mid-gestation, an episode of 12 hours' hypoxaemia is enough to cause white matter damage and neuronal death in the hippocampus, cerebral cortex and cerebellum.[29]

## INTRAPARTUM COMPLICATIONS PLAY AN INFREQUENT ROLE IN THE CAUSATION OF CEREBRAL PALSY

If a fetus has suffered neurological damage or mal-development during pregnancy, the neurological lesions, which are often multifocal, may affect parts of the fetal brain responsible for the autonomic nervous system that control such activities as heart rate and respiration. Reduced variability of the fetal heart rate, meconium staining seen at membrane rupture, low Apgar scores and neonatal encephalopathy may all represent the first recognised signs of chronic neurological compromise. In a chronically compromised case, the intrapartum signs may precipitate an obstetric intervention, such as an instrumental or Caesarean delivery, in the vain hope that the pathology is of recent onset and still reversible. Retrospectively, the presence of these signs and the decision of the carers to act to prevent possible acute compromise may mistakenly be taken as evidence of acute compromise.

It is not currently possible to recognise the point at which cerebral damage becomes irreversible in the case of an intermittent type of fetal asphyxia or intra-uterine growth restriction (IUGR). It is possible that the point of irreversible neurological injury could be reached in labour if the fetus has been able to compensate adequately until that time. IUGR of potential pathological significance can be difficult to detect clinically and randomised trials are awaited to see if earlier delivery, when moderate to severe IUGR is suspected,

**Table 7.1** Criteria to define an acute intrapartum hypoxic event

**Essential criteria**

1. Evidence of a metabolic acidosis in intrapartum fetal, umbilical arterial cord or very early neonatal blood samples. pH < 7.00 and base deficit ≥ 12 mMol/l.

2. Early onset of severe or moderate neonatal encephalopathy in infants ≥ 34 weeks' gestation.

3. Cerebral palsy is of the spastic quadriplegic or dyskinetic type.

Criteria that together suggest an intrapartum timing but by themselves are non-specific

4. A sentinel (signal) hypoxic event occurring immediately before or during labour.

5. A sudden, rapid and sustained deterioration of the fetal heart rate pattern usually following the hypoxic sentinel event where the pattern was previously normal.

6. Apgar scores of 0–6 for longer than 5 min.

7. Early evidence of multi-system involvement.

8. Early imaging evidence of acute cerebral abnormality.

reduces the incidence of cerebral palsy without a greater increase in the complications of prematurity.[30,31]

## CRITERIA SUGGESTING THAT ACUTE INTRAPARTUM HYPOXIA WAS THE CAUSE OF CEREBRAL PALSY

Table 7.1 shows the template of evidence required to suggest the occurrence of damaging intrapartum hypoxia sufficient to cause permanent neurological impairment. Taken together, criteria 4–8 help to time the hypoxic event to the intrapartum period.

## UNAVAILABLE OR CONTRARY EVIDENCE

All three of the essential criteria are necessary before an intrapartum hypoxic cause of cerebral palsy can begin to be considered. If any one of the essential criteria is not met, it strongly suggests that intrapartum hypoxia was not the cause of the cerebral palsy. If blood gas data are not available, it cannot be assumed from other signs that hypoxia was present at birth since these signs lack specificity either individually or as a group.[32–34] When all three essential criteria are met, it is then necessary to determine whether the hypoxia was acute or chronic. If evidence for some of criteria 4–8 is missing or contradictory, the timing of the onset of the neuropathology becomes increasingly in doubt. Individually, these latter criteria are only weakly associated with an acute intrapartum damaging hypoxic event because, with the exception of criterion 4 (a sentinel hypoxic event), they may be caused by other factors such as infection.[5] Logically, most of the final five criteria would have to be present for the balance of probabilities to suggest an acute timing to the hypoxic event. Contrary evidence, rather than missing evidence (e.g. a normal Apgar score at 5 min) would weigh against a serious acute event.

## COMMENTS ON PROPOSED CRITERIA

### METABOLIC ACIDAEMIA

Although its presence does not define the timing of its onset, metabolic acidaemia at birth will have to be present if a potentially damaging intrapartum hypoxic event is postulated. However, metabolic acidaemia at birth is relatively common (2% of all births) and the vast majority of such infants do not develop cerebral palsy.[35]

A realistic cut-off point for defining pathological fetal acidaemia that correlates with an increasing risk of neurological deficit has been found to be pH < 7.00 and a base deficit of >16 mMol/l.[36,37] These are also the criteria agreed by the Society of Obstetricians and Gynaecologists of Canada[13] and the American College of Obstetricians and Gynecologists.[12] It is unlikely that acute acidosis of lesser severity under these levels could be directly associated with cerebral palsy. However, occasional cases have been reported where the base deficit has been in the range of 12–15 mMol/l and thus an arterial base deficit of less than 12 mMol/l is a reasonable exclusion criterion.[38] If fetal, cord or very early (< 1 h) neonatal blood gas evidence does not exist, it is not possible to say that hypoxia or asphyxia caused or contributed to the other clinical signs. If records of both arterial and venous umbilical cord gases exist, then a difference in $PCO_2$ of > 25 mmHg suggests an acute rather than chronic acidosis.[39] However, the technique for measuring arterial versus venous gases is critical.[40] Individual $PO_2$ levels are not helpful in this context as they correlate poorly with fetal acidosis.[39] A metabolic acidosis measured in the neonate can also reflect neonatal asphyxial exposure attributable to difficult resuscitation and thus neonatal gas results carry less weight in determining an intrapartum cause.

### NEONATAL ENCEPHALOPATHY

If an intrapartum insult has caused permanent brain damage in an infant above 34 weeks of gestation, there will be abnormalities of behaviour in the neonatal period, usually of at least moderate severity and noted within 24 h of delivery. However, moderate to severe encephalopathy following a non-reassuring intrapartum cardiotocograph is very uncommon at 7 per 1000, i.e. just twice the rate in the background population.[41] Conversely, many cases of severe neonatal encephalopathy are not associated with intrapartum hypoxaemia.[17–20] Cerebral palsy associated with intrapartum events in infants born beyond 34 weeks' gestation, is only rarely an outcome associated with milder grades of encephalopathy.[42–44] Infants with severe encephalopathy frequently have an adverse outcome.[42] The outcome of those with moderate encephalopathy is less certain. The Sarnat grades[45] of encephalopathy are commonly used, but there are some differences in opinion about the criteria defining moderate and severe encephalopathy.[16] There is difficulty, short of the presence of seizure activity, in defining neonatal encephalopathy in infants below 34 weeks at birth, where many of the diagnostic criteria described in near-term infants would be part of the normal preterm course before 34 weeks (e.g. difficulty initiating and maintaining respiration, abnormal tone and feeding difficulties). Because of this and the absence of clear evidence in the literature, we can be less definite on the link between abnormal newborn behavioural states in the preterm infant and cerebral palsy attributable to an intrapartum aetiology.

## CEREBRAL PALSY TYPE

Spastic quadriplegia and, less commonly, dyskinetic cerebral palsy are the only subtypes of cerebral palsy associated with acute hypoxic intrapartum events.[42,46] Spastic quadriplegia is not specific to intrapartum hypoxia. Only 24% of a population based series of children with moderate or severe spastic quadriplegia were thought possibly, or very likely, to have been affected by intrapartum events.[46] Hemiplegic cerebral palsy, spastic diplegia and ataxia have not been associated with acute intrapartum hypoxia. This is true also for intellectual disability, autism and learning disorder in a child without spasticity. Any progression of neurological disability is not cerebral palsy by definition and is most unlikely to be secondary to birth events. Many conditions likely to be confused with cerebral palsy (e.g. Rett syndrome and Angelman syndrome) should be excluded.[47]

## SENTINEL HYPOXIC EVENT

The healthy fetus has many special physiological mechanisms to protect it from recurrent transient mild hypoxic episodes that can occur during labour.[48] For a neurologically intact fetus, uncompromised by chronic hypoxia, to sustain a neurologically damaging acute hypoxia, a serious pathological sentinel hypoxic event has to occur. Examples are ruptured uterus, placental abruption, cord prolapse, amniotic fluid embolism and fetal exsanguination from vasa previa or fetal-maternal haemorrhage. An antepartum or intrapartum hypoxic event can be silent. It is only when it is apparent or detectable that it helps define the probable timing of the event and the determination of whether its sequelae might have been preventable.

## FETAL HEART RATE

What little randomised controlled evidence as is available suggests that use of electronic fetal monitoring does not prevent cerebral palsy.[49] Even the electronic fetal monitoring observations most associated with cerebral palsy, i.e. multiple late decelerations and decreased beat-to-beat variability, should not be used to predict cerebral palsy as they have a false positive rate of

99.8%.[50] Pre-existing neurological defects may cause a reduction or absence of fetal heart variability. The high frequency (up to 79%) of non-reassuring patterns on electronic monitoring of normal pregnancies in labour with normal fetal outcomes makes both the decision on the optimal management of the labour and the prediction of current or future neurological status of the fetus very difficult.[51] Retrospective analysis of fetal heart rate traces where the neonatal outcome is known by the reviewer significantly biases obstetricians who are asked to judge the appropriateness of care.[52] Fetal heart rate patterns of potential severe fetal compromise merit early delivery where this can be achieved without undue risk to the health and life of the mother.

This Task Force endorses the statement by the US National Institute of Child Health and Human Development on electronic fetal monitoring,[53] which presented recommendations for standardised definitions of each of the characteristics of the fetal heart rate pattern. The North American Committee had a great deal of difficulty in reaching consensus on appropriate management of certain heart rate patterns, except for two. The first is that in the case of the fetus with a baseline heart rate within the normal range, 110–160 bpm and moderate FHR variability (6–25 bpm) and absent decelerations, the fetus was not at risk of acidaemia. The Committee also stated that, at the other extreme of fetal heart rate patterns, a fetus demonstrating absent fetal heart rate variability in the presence of persistent late or variable decelerations, or a bradycardia, had evidence of potentially damaging acidaemia. The Committee further decided that, because of insufficient evidence, it was impossible at this stage to reach consensus on the management of all other patterns that are variants of the normal pattern. Such recommendations will have to await further research on the reliability, validity and ability of monitoring as a means of avoiding adverse outcomes by prompting obstetric action.

## APGAR SCORES

Apgar scoring is a quick and somewhat subjective method of assessing the condition of the newborn. Low Apgar scores do not indicate the cause of the poor condition as they may result from many different factors, of which acute intrapartum hypoxia is only one. By themselves, Apgar scores are poor predictors of neurological outcome. In particular, in the preterm infant, the Apgar score is highly limited in this respect.[54] While the risk of poor outcome increases with decreasing Apgar score and increasing duration of low scores, a 5 min Apgar score below 4 but improving thereafter was associated with an increase in the risk of cerebral palsy from 0.3% to only 1% for births > 2.5 kg in the 1950s and 1960s.[55] Currently, duration of low Apgar scores is more likely to indicate the effectiveness of resuscitation than to predict outcome.[56]

## MULTI-SYSTEM INVOLVEMENT

Multi-system involvement may include acute bowel necrosis, renal failure, hepatic injury, cardiac damage, respiratory complications or haematological insult.[57–59] This requires testing over the early neonatal period (within 24 h).

Acute hypoxia usually affects all the vital organs and not just the brain, but may occasionally occur without major dysfunction of other organs.[60]

## NEONATAL BRAIN IMAGING

Early cerebral oedema, with or without intracerebral haemorrhage, suggests recent morbidity. After an acute cerebral insult, oedema appears within 6–12 h and clears by 4 days post insult.[61] Macroscopic abnormalities suggesting long-standing neurological changes may be visualised, but dysfunction which is at an intracellular level will be missed. MRI is currently the most informative imaging modality, but requires the greatest resources and is not widely available in many countries.[62] Although it may usefully predict future neurological disability in the neonate or infant, MRI has not yet been validated (against well-defined and -timed acute fetal asphyxial events) as a retrospective tool reliably defining the timing of the initial or main neuropathological event. Neonatal ultrasound evidence is more often available but false-positive and false-negative results are possible.[63] Cerebral haemorrhage and oedema can also occur later in the neonatal period, in which case it is not the result of acute intrapartum hypoxia.

## EVIDENCE FOR POSSIBLE ANTENATAL CAUSES OF CEREBRAL PALSY

Possible antenatal causes of neurological impairment are listed in Table 7.2. The presence of any one of these factors greatly reduces the likelihood that acute intrapartum hypoxia was the cause, or the sole cause, of any subsequent neurological impairment. The absence of any of these factors does not exclude an antenatal cause, as much of the evidence can be very difficult to ascertain retrospectively.

## TESTS AND SIGNS OF LESS PREDICTIVE VALUE

### MECONIUM STAINING OF AMNIOTIC FLUID

It is not possible reliably, either by inspection or by placental histopathology, to distinguish clearly between old and fresh meconium staining of amniotic fluid, nor to date the time interval between meconium passage and birth. Oligo-hydramnios will increase the concentration of any meconium in the amniotic fluid. Oligohydramnios may be associated with intra-uterine growth restriction.

### PLACENTAL PATHOLOGY AND THE TIMING OF HYPOXIC-ISCHAEMIC CEREBRAL INJURY

At present there are few methodologically rigorous studies to link various forms of chronic placental pathology and long-term neurodevelopmental

**Table 7.2** Factors that suggest a cause of cerebral palsy other than acute intrapartum hypoxia

1. Umbilical arterial base deficit < 12 mMol/l or pH > 7.00.

2. Infants with major or multiple congenital or metabolic abnormalities.

3. Central nervous system or systemic infection.

4. Early imaging evidence of long-standing neurological abnormalities (e.g. ventriculomegaly, porencephaly, multicystic encephalomalacia).

5. Infants with signs of intra-uterine growth restriction.

6. Reduced fetal heart rate variability from the onset of labour.

7. Microcephaly at birth (head circumference < 3rd percentile).

8. Major antenatal placental abruption.

9. Extensive chorio-amnionitis.

10. Congenital coagulation disorders in the child.

11. Presence of other major antenatal risk factors for cerebral palsy (e.g. preterm birth < 34 weeks gestation, multiple pregnancy, autoimmune disease).

12. Presence of major postnatal risk factors for cerebral palsy (e.g. postnatal encephalitis, prolonged hypotension or hypoxia due to severe respiratory disease).

13. A sibling with cerebral palsy especially of the same type.

outcomes despite numerous studies of candidate lesions.[64] Recent suggestions that thrombosis in large fetal vessels in the placenta can be linked to ischaemic cerebral lesions and cerebral palsy merit further investigations in appropriately designed studies of adequate size.[65,66] However, it would be unjustifiable to conclude that the absence in any particular case of any of the chronic placental lesions which, by their nature could reasonably be assumed to have antedated labour, necessarily means that an hypoxic injury must have occurred during labour.

## IN CASES OF EXCESSIVE INTRAPARTUM HYPOXIA ARE THE NEUROLOGICAL SEQUELAE PREVENTABLE?

It is not possible to ascertain retrospectively whether earlier obstetric intervention could have prevented cerebral damage in any individual case where no detectable sentinel hypoxic event occurred. Following a detectable sentinel hypoxic event, it is necessary to consider the local conditions and facilities available at the time of the birth in question when commenting whether the care provided met acceptable standards. Any major deviations from the range of normal clinical responses can only be considered critical to the development of cerebral palsy if they could plausibly and most likely have affected the duration or severity of the hypoxic event(s). The actual length of time and degree of hypoxia required to produce cerebral palsy in a previously healthy human fetus is not known. There are many special physiological mechanisms that protect the fetus from acute hypoxia allowing it to survive intact, for a longer period of minutes and perhaps hours, than an adult with

**Table 7.3** Questions pertinent to assessing the preventability of cerebral palsy assumed to be due to an acute intrapartum event

1. Were there risk factors for an antenatal cause of cerebral palsy?

2. Was there a sentinel hypoxic event?

3. Was there an intervention available proven to reduce the rate of cerebral palsy?[68]

4. Have the criteria for defining an acute intrapartum hypoxic event been met?

5. Could the signs of fetal compromise reasonably have been detected?

6. Was there an avoidable major delay in expediting delivery?

7. Would quicker delivery of the baby have compromised the mother's health or life?

8. Would an earlier delivery, if practical, have prevented or ameliorated the outcome?

similar blood gas levels.[48]. The questions in Table 7.3 should be posed when trying to identify possibly preventable causes of cerebral palsy during pregnancy, labour and delivery. Standards of care should be dictated by systematic review of high quality research.[67]

## WHO SHOULD BE AN EXPERT WITNESS IN CEREBRAL PALSY CASES?

No one person is an expert in all the facets of cerebral palsy. This Task Force has, therefore, drawn on a wide variety of disciplines for contributions to this

**Table 7.4** Recommendations for expert witnesses giving evidence on cerebral palsy causation

**Choice of witness**

1. The witness must have full qualifications in the area in which he/she is giving an opinion.

2. The witness must have credibility with respect to his/her knowledge among his/her peers, proven, for example, by relevant research published in peer-reviewed journals, ongoing continuing education and quality assurance activities.

3. In most circumstances, the witness should still be practising in that area, show evidence of being familiar with the current relevant literature and have a reasonable understanding of the local conditions and facilities at the time of the birth in question.

**Conduct of witness**

4. The witness should avoid giving specific opinions outside of his/her expertise.

5. Experts should advise: (i) of the spectrum of care considered reasonable by their profession at the time of the birth; and (ii) of all the options in any clinical situation rather than only of the ideal option in the best of circumstances with the advantage of hindsight.

6. An expert should not be an advocate for either party, but should advise and educate on the scientific and clinical validity or otherwise of the evidence.

Statement. Clearly, experts should keep to their own true area of expertise.[68] They should not be tempted to offer opinions in areas where they are not qualified to do so.[69] A peer in obstetrics is the best person to assess the clinical management of an obstetrician and a neonatologist the neonatal management. A variety of evidence-based opinions may be needed to elucidate further the possible causes of cerebral palsy in a particular case.[70]. The appropriate eligibility criteria to offer expert medico-legal clinical opinion in regard to cerebral palsy are detailed in Table 7.4.

## CONCLUSION

This International Consensus Statement has been prepared to help the public, health care workers, those researching in this area and, where necessary, courts of law to understand more easily the probability of whether, in any particular case, there is convincing evidence to suggest that the pathology causing cerebral palsy occurred during labour and whether it was reasonably preventable. Recent research strongly suggests that the large majority of neurological pathologies causing cerebral palsy occur as a result of multifactorial and mostly unpreventable reasons during fetal development or during the neonatal period.

## ACKNOWLEDGEMENT

This chapter is published with the permission of the Editor of the *British Medical Journal* where it first appeared on 16 October 1999.

### References

1 Stanley F, Alberman E. The Epidemiology of the Cerebral Palsies. Philadelphia, PA: JB Lippincott, 1984

2 Nelson KB, Ellenberg JH. Antecedents of cerebral palsy. Multivariate analysis of risk. N Engl J Med 1986; 315: 81–86

3 Volpe JJ. Metabolic encephalopathies. In: Volpe JJ. Neurology of the Newborn. Philadelphia, PA: Saunders, 1995; 467–582

4 Nelson KB, Dambrosia JM, Grether JK, Phillips TM. Neonatal cytokines and coagulation factors in children with cerebral palsy. Ann Neurol 1998; 44: 665–675

5 Grether JK, Nelson KB. Maternal infection and cerebral palsy in infants of normal birth weight. JAMA 1997; 278: 207–211

6 Nelson KB, Grether JK. Potentially asphyxiating conditions and spastic cerebral palsy in infants of normal birth weight. Obstet Gynecol 1998; 179: 507–513

7 Evrard P, Gadisseux J, Gressens P. Hypoxia opportunism during brain development. In: Wright LL, Merenstein GB, Hirtz D. (eds) Acute Perinatal Asphyxia in Term Infants. Bethesda, MD: National Institute of Child Health and Human Development, NIH, 1996; 43–50

8 Blair E, Stanley FJ. Intrapartum asphyxia: a rare cause of cerebral palsy. J Pediatr 1988; 112: 515–519

9 Blair E, Stanley F. When can cerebral palsy be prevented? The generation of causal hypotheses by mutivariate analysis of a case-control study. Paediatr Perinat Epidemiol 1993; 7: 272–301

10 Nelson KB. Relationship of intrapartum and delivery room events to long-term neurologic outcome. Clin Perinat 1989; 16: 995–1007

11 The Australian and New Zealand Perinatal Societies. The origins of cerebral palsy – a consensus statement. Med J Aust 1995; 162: 85–90

12  ACOG Committee on Obstetric Practice. Inappropriate use of the terms fetal distress and birth asphyxia. Washington DC: American College of Obstetricians and Gynecologists, 1998; Opinion 197

13  Society of Obstetricians and Gynaecologists of Canada Task Force on cerebral palsy and fetal asphyxia. J Soc Obstet Gynaecol Can 1996; 18: 1267–1279

14  Low JA. Intrapartum fetal asphyxia: definition, diagnosis and classification. Am J Obstet Gynecol 1997; 176: 957–959

15  Bax M, Nelson KB. Birth asphyxia; a statement. Dev Med Child Neurol 1993; 35: 1022–1024

16  Leviton A, Nelson KB. Problems with definitions and classifications of newborn encephalopathy. Pediatr Neurol 1992; 8: 85–90

17  Nelson KB, Leviton A. How much of neonatal encephalopathy is due to birth asphyxia? Am J Dis Child 1991; 145: 1325–1331

18  Adamson SJ, Alessandri LM, Badawi N, Burton PR, Pemberton PJ, Stanley F. Predictors of neonatal encephalopathy in full-term infants. BMJ 1995; 311: 598–602

19  Badawi N, Kurinczuk JJ, Keogh JM et al. Antepartum risk factors for newborn encephalopathy: The Western Australian Case Control Study. BMJ 1998; 317: 1549–1553

20  Badawi N, Kurinczuk JJ, Keogh JM et al. Intrapartum risk factors for newborn encephalopathy: The Western Australian Case Control Study. BMJ 1998; 317: 1554–1558

21  Yudkin PL, Johnson A, Clover LM, Murphy KW. Assessing the contribution of birth asphyxia to cerebral palsy in term singletons. Paediatr Perinat Epidemiol 1995; 9: 156–170

22  Nelson K. What proportion of cerebral palsy is related to birth asphyxia? J Pediatr 1988; 112: 572–574

23  Blair E, Stanley F. Intrauterine growth and spastic cerebral palsy. I. Association with birth weight for gestational age. Am J Obstet Gynecol 1990; 162: 229–237

24  Naeye R, Peters E, Bartholomew M, Landis JR. The origins of cerebral palsy. Am J Dis Child 1989; 143: 1154–1161

25  Nelson KB, Ellenberg JH. Obstetric complications as risk factors for cerebral palsy or seizure disorders. JAMA 1984; 251: 1843–1848

26  Nelson KB, Emery ES. Birth asphyxia and the neonatal brain: what do we know and when do we know it? Clin Perinat 1993; 20: 327–344

27  Soothill PW, Nicolaides K, Campbell S. Prenatal asphyxia, hyperlacticaemia, hypogly-caemia and erythroblastosis in growth retarded fetuses. BMJ 1987; 294: 1051–1053

28  Mallard EC, Rees S, Stringer M, Cock ML, Harding R. Effects of chronic placental insufficiency on brain development in fetal sheep. Pediatr Res 1998; 43: 262–270

29  Rees S, Mallard C, Breen S, Stringer M, Cock M, Harding R. Fetal brain injury following prolonged hypoxemia and placental insufficiency: a review. Comp Biochem Physiol 1998; 119: 653–660

30  The Growth Restriction Intervention Trial Study Group. When do obstetricians recommend delivery for a high risk pre-term growth-retarded fetus? The GRIT Study Group. Eur J Obstet Gynecol Reprod Biol 1996; 67: 121–126

31  Manning FA, Bondaji N, Harman CR et al. Fetal assessment based on fetal biophysical profile scoring. VIII. The incidence of cerebral palsy in tested and untested perinates. Am J Obstet Gynecol 1998; 178: 696–706

32  Freeman JM, Nelson KB. Intrapartum asphyxia and cerebral palsy. Pediatrics 1988; 82: 240–249

33  Perlman JM. Intrapartum hypoxic-ischemic cerebral injury and subsequent cerebral palsy: medico-legal issues. Pediatrics 1997; 99: 851–859

34  van der Riet JE, Vandenbussche FP, Le Cessie S, Keirse MJNC. Newborn assessment and long-term adverse outcome: a systemic review. Am J Obstet Gynecol 1999; 180: 1024–1029

35  Ruth VJ, Raivio KO. Perinatal brain damage: predictive value of metabolic acidosis and the Apgar score. BMJ 1988; 297: 24–27

36  Goldaber GK, Gilstrap III LC, Levono KJ, Dax JS, McIntyre DD. Pathologic fetal acidemia. Obstet Gynecol 1991; 78; 1103–1111

37  Sehdev HM, Stamilio DM, Macones GA, Graham E, Morgan MA. Predictive factors for neonatal morbidity in neonates with an umbilical cord pH less than 7.00. Am J Obstet Gynecol 1997; 177: 1030–1034

38 Low JA, Lindsay BG, Derrick EJ. Threshold of metabolic acidosis associated with newborn complications. Am J Obstet Gynecol 1997; 177: 1391–1394

39 Belai YI, Goodwin TM, Durand M, Greenspoon JP, Paul RH, Walther FJ. Umbilical arteriovenous $PO_2$ and $PCO_2$ differences and neonatal morbidity in term infants with severe acidosis. Am J Obstet Gynecol 1998; 178: 13–19

40 Westgate J, Garibaldi JM, Greene KR. Umbilical cord blood gas analysis at delivery: a time for quality data. Br J Obstet Gynaecol 1994; 101: 1054–1063

41 Spencer JA, Badawi N, Burton B, Keogh J, Pemberton P, Stanley F. The intrapartum CTG prior to neonatal encephalopathy at term: a case-control study. Br J Obstet Gynaecol 1997; 104: 25–28

42 Rosenbloom L. Dyskinetic cerebral palsy and birth asphyxia. Dev Med Child Neurol 1994; 36: 285–289

43 Robertson CM, Finer NN. Long-term follow-up of term neonates with perinatal asphyxia. Clin Perinat 1993; 20: 483–500

44 Nelson KB, Ellenberg JH. The asymptomatic newborn and risk of cerebral palsy. Am J Dis Child 1987; 141: 1333–1335

45 Sarnat HB, Sarnat MS. Neonatal encephalopathy following fetal distress. A clinical and electroencephalographic study. Arch Neurol 1976; 33: 696–705

46 Stanley FJ, Blair E, Hockey A, Petterson B, Watson L. Spastic quadriplegia in Western Australia: a genetic epidemiological study. Dev Med Child Neurol 1993; 35: 191–201

47 Badawi N, Watson L, Petterson B et al. What constitutes cerebral palsy? Dev Med Child Neurol 1998; 40: 520–527

48 Meschia G. Placental respiratory gas exchange and fetal oxygenation. In: Creasy RK, Resnik R. (eds) Maternal Fetal Medicine Principles and Practice. Philadelphia, PA: Saunders, 1994; 288–297

49 Grant A, O'Brien N, Joy M, Hennessy E, MacDonald D. Cerebral palsy among children born during the Dublin randomised trial of intrapartum monitoring. Lancet 1989; ii: 1233–1236

50 Nelson KB, Dambrosia JM, Ting TY, Grether JK. Uncertain value of electronic fetal monitoring in predicting cerebral palsy. N Engl J Med 1996; 334: 613–618

51 Umstad MP, Permezel M, Pepperell RJ. Intrapartum cardiotocography and the expert witness. Aust N Z J Obstet Gynaecol 1994; 34: 20–23

52 Zain HA, Wright JW, Parrish GE, Diehl SJ. Interpreting the fetal heart rate tracing. Effect of knowledge of the neonatal outcome. J Reprod Med 1998; 43: 367–370

53 National Institute of Child Health and Human Development Research Planning Workshop. Electronic fetal heart rate monitoring: research guidelines for interpretation. Am J Obstet Gynecol 1997; 177: 1385–1390

54 Topp M, Langhoff-Roos J, Uldall P. Preterm birth and cerebral palsy. Predictive value of pregnancy complications, mode of delivery and Apgar scores. Acta Obstet Gynecol Scand 1997; 76: 843–848

55 Nelson KB, Ellenberg JH. Apgar scores as predictors of chronic neurologic disability. Pediatrics 1981; 68: 36–44

56 Committee on Fetus and Newborn, American Academy of Pediatrics, and Committee on Obstetric Practice, American College of Obstetricians and Gynecologists. Use and abuse of the Apgar Score. Pediatrics 1996; 98: 141–142

57 Perlman JM, Tack EC, Martin T, Shackelford G, Amon E. Acute systemic organ injury in term infants after asphyxia. Am J Dis Child 1989; 143: 617–620

58 Willis F, Summers J, Minutillo C, Hewitt I. Indices of renal tubular function in perinatal asphyxia. Arch Dis Child Fetal Neonatal Ed 1997; 77: F57–F60

59 Martinancel A, Garciaalix A, Gaya F, Cabanas F, Burgueros M, Quero J. Multiple organ involvement in perinatal asphyxia. J Pediatr 1995; 127: 786–793

60 Phelan JP, Ahn MO, Korst L, Martin GI, Wang YM. Intrapartum fetal asphyxial brain injury with absent multiorgan system dysfunction. J Matern Fetal Med 1998; 7: 19–22

61 Govaert P, de Vries LS. An atlas of neonatal brain sonography. Clin Dev Med 1997; 244: 141–142

62 Barkovich AJ, Hajnal BL, Vigneron D et al. Prediction of neuro-motor outcome in perinatal asphyxia – evaluation of MR scoring systems. Am J Neuroradiol 1998; 19: 143–149

63 Barkovich AJ. The encephalopathic neonate – choosing the proper imaging technique. Am J Neuroradiol 1997; 18: 1816–1820

64 Grafe MR. The correlation of prenatal brain damage with placental pathology. J Neuropathol Exp Neurol 1994; 53: 407–415

65 Kraus FT. Cerebral palsy and thrombi in placental vessels of the fetus: insights from litigation. Hum Pathol 1997; 28: 246–248

66 Burke JC, Tannenberg AE, Payton DJ. Ischaemic cerebral injury, intrauterine growth retardation and placental infarction. Dev Med Child Neurol 1997; 39: 726–730

67 Stanley F, Blair E, Alberman E. Possibilities for the prevention of the cerebral palsies: social and medical. Clin Dev Med 2000; 151: 138–175

68 Medico-legal Committee of the Society of Obstetrics and Gynaecologists of Canada. The expert witness. J Soc Obstet Gynaecol Can 1997; 19: 296–306

69 Fisher CW, Dombrowski MP, Jaszczak SE, Cook CD, Sokol RJ. The expert witness: real issues and suggestions. Am J Obstet Gynecol 1995; 172: 1792–1800

70 Samuels G. Medical truth and legal proof. Changing expectations of the expert witness. Med J Aust 1998; 168: 84–87

*Andrew Prentice*

# Advances in the management of endometriosis related infertility

The implementation of evidence-based medicine provides us with the opportunity to practice medicine based on the best available evidence. The perception exists, however, that evidence-based medicine is restricted to answering therapeutic questions such as: 'is A a suitable treatment for condition X?' or 'is A better than B in the treatment of condition Y?' Evidence-based medicine goes beyond these important considerations and allows the application of rational treatments based upon a sound understanding of the underlying pathophysiology. In the management of infertility related to endometriosis, this is pertinent. In some cases the causal relationship between endometriosis and infertility is clear, but in other cases, particularly with minimal disease, the relationship is less apparent. An understanding of the mechanisms by which the reduction in the fertility occurs and the correction of that abnormality is the most logical and rational management strategy. In this chapter, the putative mechanisms by which endometriosis causes infertility will be examined and the management of patients with infertility associated with early and late stage endometriosis.

## MECHANISM OF INFERTILITY IN ENDOMETRIOSIS

Endometriosis at all stages is associated with a reduction in conception rates.[1] With advanced disease, the destruction of the normal anatomy may interfere with normal spatial relationships between the Fallopian tubes and ovaries. Consequently, the disease process may interfere with ovarian mobility, oocyte release, oocyte pick up, and tubal motility and patency. With less advanced disease, no such obvious relationship exists and many putative mechanisms have been suggested.

**Mr Andrew Prentice** BSc MA MD MRCOG, Consultant Gynaecologist and University Lecturer, Department of Obstetrics and Gynaecology, University of Cambridge, Box 223 The Rosie Hospital, Robinson Way, Cambridge CB2 2SW, UK

Putative mechanisms of infertility fall into three broad groups: (i) disorders of folliculogenesis or endocrine abnormality; (ii) inflammatory or immunological abnormality; and (iii) increased miscarriage rate. A number of authors have reviewed the literature and report no convincing evidence of either an abnormality of follicular development or an endocrine abnormality that explains infertility in all cases of endometriosis.[2,3] Endocrine abnormalities have been reported, but no evidence that they are more common in women with endometriosis than in other infertile women or that they occur consistently in consecutive cycles.

In a disease where the fundamental abnormality was endometrial, an increased failure of implantation would be expected. This would manifest as a higher incidence of early pregnancy loss. Early retrospective cohort studies of endometriosis reported miscarriage rates in excess of 40%.[4,5] Pittaway and colleagues,[6] in a prospective study, showed that other explanations for miscarriage existed and that, similar to infertile women, women with higher miscarriage rates may have visible endometriosis as a consequence of not having had an on-going pregnancy. Experience from assisted reproduction, where the early diagnosis of pregnancy allows accurate quantification of the miscarriage rate, confirms that a history of endometriosis does not result in a higher rate of early pregnancy loss.[7,8]

Patients with endometriosis have an altered peritoneal environment in the pelvis which goes beyond the visible presence of implants of ectopic endometrium. The pelvic organs are bathed in peritoneal fluid containing cellular and non-cellular components, which may effect fertility. The potential mechanisms effecting fertility are listed in Table 8.1. Whether these alterations are the cause or the consequence of the ectopic endometrium is uncertain.

In patients with endometriosis, an increased volume of peritoneal fluid has been observed throughout the menstrual cycle.[9,10] However, other studies have failed to confirm these findings.[11] The amount of peritoneal fluid may correlate with the likelihood of achieving a pregnancy; Syrop and Halme demonstrated that women who achieved pregnancy had lower peritoneal fluid volumes than those who did not.[12] Peritoneal fluid volume alone is unlikely to be the only explanation for infertility associated with early disease and medical treatment which reduces peritoneal fluid volume[13] does not improve fecundity (Fig. 8.1).[14]

The peritoneal fluid in women with endometriosis has an increase in leukocytes and 85% are macrophages.[15] The increased number of macrophages may be less important than their activation status. The proportion of activated macrophages is increased in infertile women with endometriosis by a factor of

**Table 8.1** Potential effects on infertility of the components of peritoneal fluid

Ovulatory function
Gamete transport
Gamete survival
Sperm–ovum interaction
Early embryo interaction within Fallopian tube
Implantation

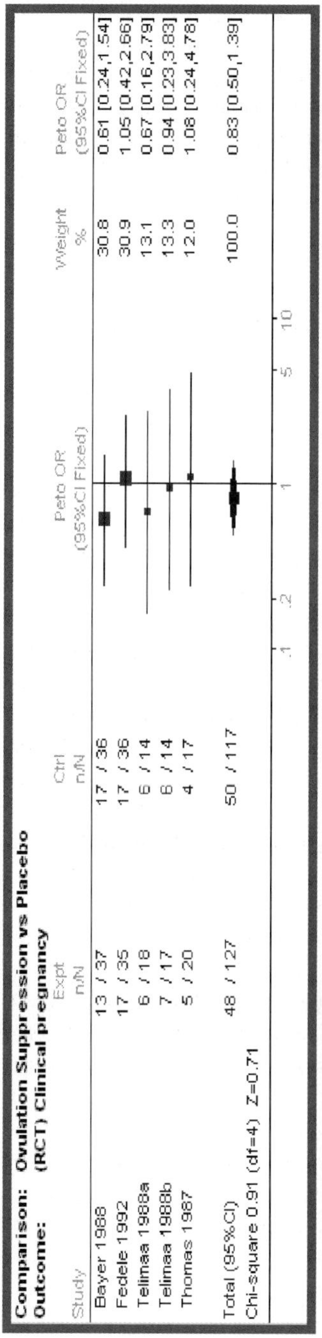

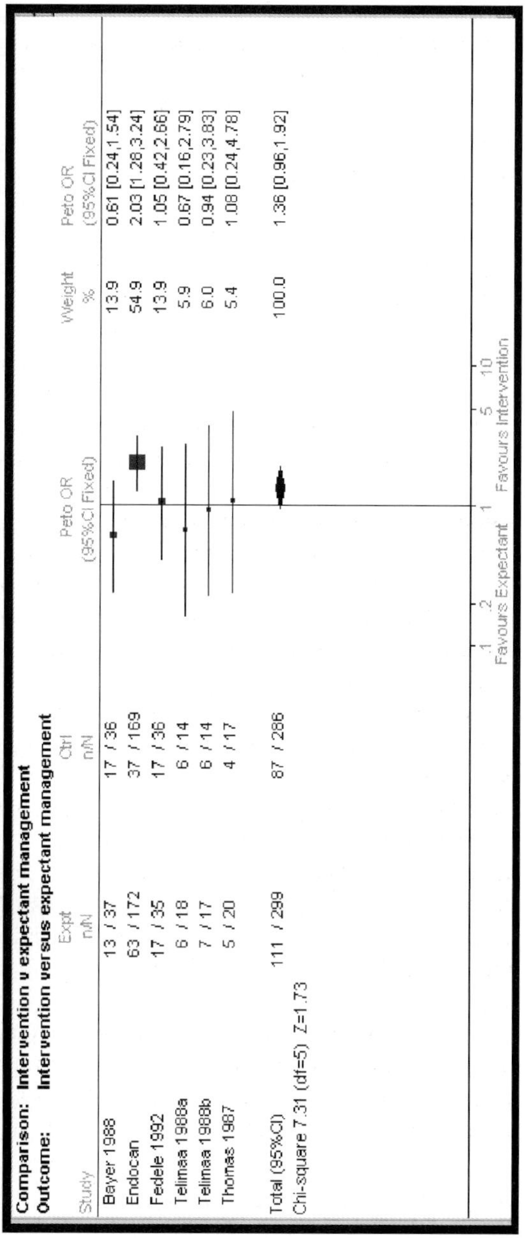

**Comparison:** Ovulation Suppression vs Placebo
**Outcome:** (RCT) Clinical pregnancy

| Study | Expt n/N | Ctrl n/N | Weight % | Peto OR (95%CI Fixed) | Peto OR (95%CI Fixed) |
|---|---|---|---|---|---|
| Bayer 1988 | 13 / 37 | 17 / 36 | 30.8 | | 0.61 [0.24,1.54] |
| Fedele 1992 | 17 / 35 | 17 / 36 | 30.9 | | 1.05 [0.42,2.66] |
| Telimaa 1988a | 6 / 18 | 6 / 14 | 13.1 | | 0.67 [0.16,2.79] |
| Telimaa 1988b | 7 / 17 | 6 / 14 | 13.3 | | 0.94 [0.23,3.83] |
| Thomas 1987 | 5 / 20 | 4 / 17 | 12.0 | | 1.08 [0.24,4.78] |
| Total (95%CI) | 48 / 127 | 50 / 117 | 100.0 | | 0.83 [0.50,1.39] |

Chi-square 0.91 (df=4) Z=0.71

**Fig. 8.1** No benefit is seen in terms of clinical pregnancy rates in suppressing ovulation in patients with endometriosis associated infertility.[14]

**Comparison:** Intervention v expectant management
**Outcome:** Intervention versus expectant management

| Study | Expt n/N | Ctrl n/N | Weight % | Peto OR (95%CI Fixed) | Peto OR (95%CI Fixed) |
|---|---|---|---|---|---|
| Bayer 1988 | 13 / 37 | 17 / 36 | 13.9 | | 0.61 [0.24,1.54] |
| Endocan | 63 / 172 | 37 / 169 | 54.9 | | 2.03 [1.28,3.24] |
| Fedele 1992 | 17 / 35 | 17 / 36 | 13.9 | | 1.05 [0.42,2.66] |
| Telimaa 1988a | 6 / 18 | 6 / 14 | 5.9 | | 0.67 [0.16,2.79] |
| Telimaa 1988b | 7 / 17 | 6 / 14 | 6.0 | | 0.94 [0.23,3.83] |
| Thomas 1987 | 5 / 20 | 4 / 17 | 5.4 | | 1.08 [0.24,4.78] |
| Total (95%CI) | 111 / 299 | 87 / 286 | 100.0 | | 1.36 [0.96,1.92] |

Chi-square 7.31 (df=5) Z=1.73

Favours Expectant — Favours Intervention

**Fig. 8.2** Meta-analysis of intervention (surgical or medical) versus expectant management in minimal and mild endometriosis.

3 (46% versus 15%)[16] and these activated macrophages may affect fertility. The mechanisms include phagocytosis of sperm by activated macrophages,[17] decreased sperm motility[18] and embryotoxicty.[19] Despite a large body of literature in this area, the precise mechanisms of infertility in early stage disease remains unclear. In clinical practice we continue to focus on the visible abnormality, the endometriotic implant.

## TREATMENT OF MINIMAL AND MILD DISEASE

### MEDICAL

A comprehensive systematic review has clearly shown that medical therapy with ovulation suppression does not improve fertility rates.[14] From the data in the trials, expected pregnancy rates with expectant management can be estimated. Pregnancy rates in the four control groups were 23.5–47.2%. Expectant management does, therefore, provide a reasonable chance of the patient achieving a pregnancy.

Medical therapy may have a role in patients with the combined problems of infertility and pain. While effective in treating pain, medical therapies have no benefit in treating infertility and their traditional use results in 6 months of contraception which further delays pregnancy. In the older age group, such a delay will further compromise the prospects of conception. In an attempt to provide medical treatment without compromising fertility, Overton et al treated patients with either 40 mg or 60 mg of dydrogesterone in the luteal phase of the cycle. Relief of symptoms was achieved without compromising fertility.[20]

### SURGICAL

The meta-analysis that confirmed the lack of efficacy of medical therapy,[14,21] also included an analysis of laparoscopic therapy. This suggested that laparoscopic surgery was more effective than either medical treatment with danazol or no treatment (odds ratio, 2.7; 95% CI, 2.1–3.5). However, the trials included were of variable methodological quality. Of the six studies, five were cohort studies and the other was a quasi-randomised study.[22] In the latter study,[22] there was no blinding of the treatment allocation and the allocation process used social security numbers. Other criticisms of this study include randomisation before laparoscopy and subsequent exclusion of patients after they had been allocated, and other interventions that could have affected outcome. Hughes and colleagues concluded that there was a need for a large randomised trial to answer the question reliably.[21]

A multi-centre randomised controlled trial was conducted in Canada.[23] The study aimed to establish whether the ablation or resection of minimal or mild endometriosis (stage I or II) improved the cumulative probability of pregnancy. The primary outcome was pregnancy progressing beyond 20 weeks' gestation. Follow-up was for 36 weeks which was longer than the 24 weeks follow-up in medical trials. The Endocan study was well designed; all other factors that might affect fertility were excluded, randomisation was at time of laparoscopy, thus avoiding the potential bias of excluding eligible women after randomisation and randomisation was performed at a distant site but patients were not blinded to randomisation. Inclusion in the study depended on the visualisation of typical blue-black endometriotic lesions and an AFS score of < 16. This unfortunately meant that patients with adhesions were included in the study and thus the intervention was not confined to ablation of implants. Another consequence of the need to identify blue-black lesions was that all cases of endometriosis may not have been included and this means that the results of the study may be limited. This may also explain the relatively low rate of the diagnosis of endometriosis in the study group. Of the 717 patients who asked to participate, only 348 (48.5%) had endometriosis diagnosed visually.

At the end of the study, 341 patients were eligible for analysis with 172 undergoing laparoscopic treatment and 169 having a diagnostic laparoscopy. Those patients undergoing laparoscopic treatment had not only an ablation of endometriotic deposits but also a division of any adhesions present. While the aim was to study the effect of ablation or resection in a proportion of patients, a significant co-intervention took place. In more than 9% of patients, other co-interventions took place which may have influenced the primary outcome. The inclusion of adhesiolysis was inevitable as patients were included if they had stage I or II disease and some patients with stage II disease will have adhesions. When surgery was performed, the vast majority (78%) were treated with electrocautery.

Patients treated at time of laparoscopy had a significantly higher pregnancy rate than those who underwent only a diagnostic laparoscopy (30.7% versus 17.7%; odds ratio, 1.7; 95% CI, 1.2–2.6). Excluding. those with adhesions, the odds ratio was still higher (1.6; 95% CI 1.2–2.5), but in both groups the confidence intervals are quite wide and the lower value approaches one. When patients with adhesions are excluded, only 284 patients remain and thus the study to consider the effect of ablation alone is under-powered as 330 patients were required. Despite a longer follow-up period than the 24 weeks used in randomised controlled trials of medical therapy, the cumulative probability of pregnancy in the treated group is less than the expectant management group of some medical trials where pregnancy rates ranged from 23.5–47.2%.[14] This again may reflect the impact of the inclusion of patients with adhesions.

Surgery may be just another way of abolishing endometriotic implants. Data from trials indicate that medical therapy can result in the complete disappearance of all endometriotic implants.[24] On this basis, we can include this trial in a meta-analysis of all treatments of endometriosis whilst accepting that such a combination of trials has significant clinical heterogeneity. This meta-analysis is shown in Figure 8.2 and demonstrates that, overall, the combination of trials demonstrates no benefit of intervention.

## SURGICAL TREATMENT OF ADVANCED DISEASE

Surgical correction of the distorted pelvic anatomy caused by endometriosis is widely accepted to improve fecundity. A number of questions arise regarding the surgical management. These questions include the mode of surgery, laparoscopy or laparotomy, whether medical treatment should be used as an adjunct to surgery either prior to or after surgery and what measures should be taken to prevent adhesion formation. Whatever the answers, the principles of infertility surgery should be applied, namely good exposure of the operative field and magnification, scrupulous haemostasis, minimal tissue handling and attention to the prevention of adhesion formation.

Laparoscopic surgery for advanced endometriosis can be extremely hazardous and should not been undertaken without appropriate training and experience. For gynaecologists without level III training, therefore, an open procedure will be more appropriate. What are the potential advantages of a laparoscopic approach? The laparoscopic approach has usually reduced morbidity and a more rapid return to full activity due to the absence of a large abdominal incision. However, are there are any advantages or disadvantages related to the primary indication and outcome of surgery, namely improvement of fertility and pregnancy?

Reduced tissue drying in the laparoscopic approach may reduce adhesions.[25] Reduced adhesion formation should be beneficial but for infertility the **only** endpoint that matters is pregnancy. Adamson and Patta[26] performed a meta-analysis of eight trials comparing laparoscopic surgery with laparotomy. None of the individual trials showed any benefit in using one rather than the other approach and the overall relative risk was 0.93 (95% CI, 0.84–1.02). These trials had considerable clinical heterogeneity with differing inclusion criteria, some with advanced endometriosis and others with early disease, and some trials included other factors affecting fertility.

The meta-analysis described above only considered pregnancy rates. The reduced morbidity associated with laparoscopic surgery and the consequent early return to full activity was not reflected in a higher or earlier pregnancy rate (Fig. 8.3).[27]

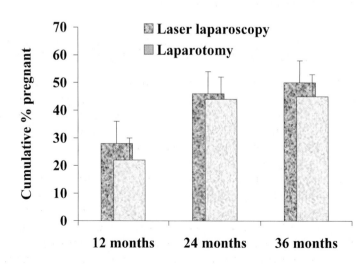

**Fig. 8.3** Cumulative pregnancy rates following infertility surgery for endometriosis. Data from Adamson et al.[27]

**Table 8.2** The effect of pre-operative medical treatment in the surgical management of moderate and severe endometriosis[29]

|  | Number pregnant | Percentage pregnant | 95% confidence interval |
|---|---|---|---|
| Surgery alone | 8/26 | 30.7 | 14–52 |
| Surgery + danazol | 7/27 | 25.9 | 11–46 |
| Surgery + MPA | 23/64 | 35.9 | 24–49 |

While surgical therapy alone is beneficial[26] and medical therapy alone offers no benefit,[14] the combination of medical and surgical therapy has to be considered. Medical therapy can be used as an adjunct either before or after surgery. Vercillini and colleagues recently published a systematic review of the role of medical therapy in all aspects of the management of endometriosis.[28] In this review, four of the eleven studies examined the use of different medical therapies: danazol (2 studies), lynestrenol (1 study), medroxyprogesterone acetate (1 study) and goserelin (1 study). Of these studies, only one considered patients whose only fertility problem was endometriosis.[29] This study compared three groups of patients with moderate or severe endometriosis treated either surgically or surgically following pre-treatment with either danazol or medroxyprogesterone acetate. The results are shown in Table 8.2 and demonstrate no significance between the groups. Vercillini and colleagues[28] performed a meta-analysis of three studies that considered postoperative medical treatment. The results of this meta-analysis demonstrated a common odds ratio of 0.72 with 95% confidence limits of 0.35 and 1.44. Thus, the addition of medical treatment as an adjunct to surgery appears to offer no additional benefit over surgery alone, just as medical therapy alone is of no benefit in treating the infertility associated with endometriosis. The failure of medical therapy to offer any benefit may reflect the fact that medical therapy, whilst relieving symptoms, does not achieve complete resolution of the implants.[30]

## ART AND ENDOMETRIOSIS

The precise relationship between infertility and endometriosis, in the absence of pelvic distortion, is unclear. Many consider the relationship to be purely casual and the patients to have unexplained infertility. Assisted reproduction techniques (ARTs) are used to treat the infertility when other treatments or expectant management have been unsuccessful. Endometriosis has been suggested as adversely effecting fertility outcomes.[8] A review of the published literature,[31] including French and US national data, does not support endometriosis having any additional adverse effect on success rates. However, doubt remains on the impact of endometriomata, the ARTs which should be employed, and the role of medical and surgical treatment prior to ART. Robinson and Hornstein[31] have suggested that a number of large, randomised controlled studies are required to determine the optimal utilisation of ART in endometriosis associated infertility. Until such studies are completed, no evidence base exists to recommend best practice.

## Key points for clinical practice

- The relationship between endometriosis and infertility in the absence of pelvic distortion remains uncertain.

- Medical treatment has little part to play in the management of endometriosis associated infertility.

- The role of surgery is both rational and established.

- In the surgical treatment of endometriosis, the laparoscope and laparotomy achieve the same cumulative pregnancy rate.

- Medical treatment as an adjunct to surgery offers no additional benefit.

- Assisted reproduction techniques have a definite place in management when other treatments have failed to resolve the problem.

### References

1 Hull MGR. The causes of infertility and relative effectiveness of treatment. In: Templeton AA, Drife JO. (eds) Infertility. London: Springer, 1992; 33–58
2 Thomas EJ. Endometriosis and infertility. In: Thomas EJ, Rock JA. (eds) Modern Approaches to Endometriosis. Dordrecht: Kluwer Academic, 1991; 113–128
3 Haney AF. Endometriosis-associated infertility. Clin Obstet Gynaecol 1993; 7: 791–812
4 Naples JD, Batt RE, Sadigh J. Spontaneous abortion rate in patients with endometriosis. Obstet Gynecol 1981; 57: 509–512
5 Olive DL, Franklin RR, Gratkins LV. The association between endometriosis and spontaneous abortion. J Reprod Med 1982; 27: 333–338
6 Pittaway DE, Vernon C, Fayez JA. Spontaneous abortion in women with endometriosis. Fertil Steril 1988; 50: 711–715
7 Geber S, Paraschos T, Atkinson G, Margara R, Winston RML. Results of IVF in patients with endometriosis: the severity of the disease does not affect outcome, or the incidence of miscarriage. Hum Reprod 1995; 10: 1507–1511
8 Omland AK, Tambo T, Dale PO et al. Artificial insemination by husband in unexplained infertility compared with infertility associated with peritoneal endometriosis. Hum Reprod 1998; 13: 2602–2605
9 Drake TS, Metz SA, Grunert GM et al. Peritoneal fluid volume in endometriosis. Fertil Steril 1980; 34: 280
10 Syrop CH, Halme J. Cyclic changes of peritoneal fluid parameters in normal and infertile patients. Obstet Gynecol 1987; 69: 416–418
11 Rezai N, Ghodgaonkar RB, Zacur HA et al. Cul-de-sac fluid in women with endometriosis: fluid volume and prostanoid concentration during the proliferative phase of the cycle days 13 to 18. Fertil Steril 1987; 48: 29–32
12 Syrop CH, Halme J. A comparison of peritoneal fluid parameters of infertile patients and the subsequent occurrence of pregnancy. Fertil Steril 1986; 46: 631–635
13 Haney AF, Weinberg JB. Reduction of the intraperitoneal inflammation associated with endometriosis by treatment with medroxyprogesterone acetate. Am J Obstet Gynecol 1988; 159: 450–454
14 Hughes E, Fedorkow D, Collins J, Vandekerckhove P. Ovulation suppression for endometriosis (Cochrane Review). In: The Cochrane Library, Issue 4. Oxford: Update Software, 1999
15 van Furth R, Raeburn JA, van Zwet TI. Characteristics of human mononuclear phagocytes. Blood 1979; 54; 485–500

16 Halme J, Becker S, Hammond MG *et al*. Increased activation of peritoneal macrophages in infertile women with endometriosis. Am J Obstet Gynecol 1983; 45: 333–337

17 Muscato JJ, Haney AF, Weinberg JB. Sperm phagocytosis by human peritoneal macrophages: a possible cause of infertility in endometriosis. Am J Obstet Gynecol 1982; 144; 503–510

18 Drudy L, Lewis SEM, Kinsella CB *et al*. The influence of peritoneal fluid from patients with minimal stage or treated endometriosis on sperm motility parameters using computer-assisted semen analysis. Hum Reprod 1994; 9; 2418–2423

19 Taketani Y, Kuo TM, Mizuno M. Comparison of cytokine levels and embryotoxicity in peritoneal fluid in infertile women with untreated or treated endometriosis. Am J Obstet Gynecol 1992; 167: 265–270

20 Overton CE, Lindsay PC, Johal B *et al*. A randomised, double-blind, placebo controlled study of luteal phase dydrogesterone (Duphaston) in women with minimal to mild endometriosis. Fertil Steril 1994; 62: 701–707

21 Hughes EG, Fedorkow, Collins JA. A quantitative overview of controlled trials in endometriosis associated infertility. Fertil Steril 1993; 93: 963–970

22 Nowroozi K, Chase JS, Check JH *et al*. The importance of laparoscopic coagulation of mild endometriosis in infertile women. Int J Fertil 1987; 87: 442–444

23 Marcoux S, Maheux R, Bérubé S and the Canadian Collaborative Group on Endometriosis. Laparoscopic surgery in infertile women with minimal and mild endometriosis. N Engl J Med 1997; 97; 212–222

24 Prentice A, Deary AJ, Goldbeck-Wood S, Farquhar C, Smith SK. Gonadotrophin-releasing hormone analogues for pain associated with endometriosis (Cochrane Review). In: The Cochrane Library, Issue 4. Oxford: Update Software, 1999

25 Nezhat CR, Nezhat FR, Metzger DA *et al*. Adhesion reformation after reproductive surgery by videolaparoscopy. Fertil Steril 1990; 53: 1008–1010

26 Adamson GD, Pasta DJ. Surgical treatment of endometriosis-associated infertility: meta-analysis compared with survival analysis. Am J Obstet Gynecol 1994; 171: 1488–1505

27 Adamson GD, Subak LL, Pasta DJ *et al*. Comparison of $CO_2$ laser laparoscopy with laparotomy for treatment of endometriomata. Fertil Steril 1992; 57: 965–973

28 Vercillini P, DeGiorgi O, Pesole A *et al*. Endometriosis: drugs and adjuvant therapy. In: Templeton A, Cooke I, O'Brien PMS. (eds) Evidence-based Fertility Treatment. London, RCOG Press, 1998; 225–245

29 Napolitano C, Marziani R, Mossa M *et al*. Management of stage III and IV endometriosis: a 10 year experience. Eur J Obstet Gynecol Reprod Biol 1994; 53: 199–204

30 Evers JLH. The second-look laparoscopy for evaluation of the result of medical treatment of endometriosis should not be performed during ovarian suppression. Fertil Steril 1987; 47: 502–504

31 Robinson RD, Hornstein RD. Effects of endometriosis on pregnancy outcome using reproductive technologies. In: Diamond MP, Osteen KG. (eds). Endometrium and Endometriosis. Malden, MA: Blackwell Science, 1997; 255–262

*Adam Balen*

# Laparoscopic treatment of polycystic ovary syndrome

This chapter will discuss laparoscopic surgery for polycystic ovary syndrome (PCOS) in the context of the treatment of anovulatory infertility. First the PCOS and the spectrum of the syndrome will be defined in order to appreciate the logistics of the alternative therapies. The PCOS is the commonest endocrine disturbance affecting women.[1] The presence of enlarged ovaries with multiple small cysts (2–8 mm) and a hypervascularized, androgen-secreting stroma has long been recognised as associated with signs of androgen excess (hirsutism, alopecia, acne), obesity and menstrual cycle disturbance (oligomenorrhoea or amenorrhoea). The European view, in general, is that the syndrome encompasses any of the above-mentioned signs, symptoms or endocrine abnormalities (elevated serum androgen and/or luteinizing hormone (LH) concentrations).[2] In North America, the consensus is that the syndrome is denoted by the combination of hyperandrogenism and ovulatory dysfunction, in the absence of non-classical adrenal hyperplasia, without necessarily having to identify the presence of polycystic ovaries by ultrasound scan.[3] The European definition, which we have designated as PCO1, is broader than that of the US (designated PCO2).

A number of interlinking factors affect ovarian function and expression of PCOS. A gain in weight is associated with a worsening of symptoms, whilst weight loss will ameliorate the endocrine and metabolic profile and symptomatology.[4] Feedback from the polycystic ovary to both the pituitary and hypothalamus appears to be disturbed due to abnormalities in the secretion of ovarian steroid hormones and – probably more important – of non-steroidal hormones, for example inhibin and related proteins.[5,6] Normal ovarian function relies upon the selection of a follicle, which responds to an appropriate signal (follicle stimulating hormone) in order to grow, become

**Mr Adam Balen** MB BS MD MRCOG, Consultant in Reproductive Medicine and Honorary Senior Lecturer, Department of Obstetrics and Gynaecology, The General Infirmary, Leeds LS2 9NS, UK

'dominant' and ovulate. This mechanism is disturbed in women with PCOS, resulting in multiple small cysts, most of which contain potentially viable oocytes but within dysfunctional follicles.

Hypersecretion of LH is found in 40% of women with PCOS and is associated with a reduced chance of conception and an increased risk of miscarriage, possibly through an adverse effect of LH on oocyte maturation.[5] Elevated serum concentrations of insulin are more common in both lean and obese women with PCOS than weight-matched controls. Indeed, hyperinsulinaemia may be the key to the pathogenesis of the syndrome.[3] Insulin stimulates androgen secretion by the ovarian stroma and appears to affect the normal development of ovarian follicles, both by the adverse effects of androgens on follicular growth and possibly also by suppressing apoptosis and permitting the survival of follicles otherwise destined to disappear.

The management of anovulatory infertility in PCOS has traditionally involved the use of clomiphene citrate and then gonadotrophin therapy or laparoscopic ovarian surgery in those who are clomiphene resistant. The principles of therapy are first to optimise health before commencing therapy (e.g. weight loss for those who are overweight) and then induce regular unifollicular ovulation, whilst minimising the risks of ovarian hyperstimulation syndrome (OHSS) and multiple pregnancy. This chapter will deal mainly with laparoscopic ovarian surgery after discussing briefly the medical alternatives.

## WEIGHT LOSS AND MEDICAL THERAPIES TO INDUCE OVULATION

Obese women (BMI > 30 kg/m$^2$), should be encouraged to lose weight. Weight loss improves the endocrine profile, the likelihood of ovulation and a healthy pregnancy.[4] Weight loss should also be encouraged prior to ovulation induction treatments, as they appear to be less effective when the BMI is greater than 28–30 kg/m$^2$.[7] The use of insulin-sensitising agents (e.g. metformin) to improve the endocrine profile, reduce weight loss and restore ovarian cyclicity is a subject of recent research,[1] but as yet cannot be recommended in routine clinical practice. Women with the PCOS who are anovulatory have traditionally been treated with anti-oestrogens (clomiphene citrate or tamoxifen) as first line therapy. Clomiphene citrate induces ovulation in approximately 70–85% of patients although only 40–50% conceive. Kousta and colleagues[8] recently reported their experience in the treatment of 167 patients and found good cumulative conception rates (67.3% over 6 months in those who had no other subfertility factors), which continued to rise up to 12 cycles of therapy. They reported a multiple pregnancy rate of 11%, similar to that described in other series and a miscarriage rate of 23.6%; those who miscarried tended to have a higher serum LH concentration immediately after clomiphene administration.

The therapeutic options for patients with anovulatory infertility who are resistant to anti-oestrogens are either parenteral gonadotrophin therapy or laparoscopic ovarian diathermy. We consider clomiphene-resistance to mean failure to ovulate (i.e. no response) while others mean failure to conceive despite ovulation (which we would call clomiphene-failure). We have published the cumulative conception and live-birth rates in 103 women with PCOS who did not ovulate with anti-oestrogen therapy.[9] While the cumulative conception and live-birth rates after 6 months were 62% and 54%, respectively, and after 12 months 73% and 62%, respectively, the rate of multiple pregnancy was 19% and there were three cases of moderate to severe ovarian hyperstimulation syndrome. We found that the rate of multiple pregnancy fell to 4% after the introduction of real-time transvaginal ultrasound monitoring of follicular development. This emphasises the central role of effective surveillance in programmes of ovulation induction. Multiple pregnancy is an undesirable side-effect of fertility therapy because of the increased rates of perinatal morbidity and mortality. In the UK, the unmonitored use of oral anti-oestrogens accounts for more cases of triplets than gonadotrophin therapy or assisted conception.[10] High order multiple pregnancies (quadruplets or more) result almost exclusively from ovulation induction therapies. It can be extremely difficult to predict the response to stimulation of women with polycystic ovaries. Gonadotrophins should be given in low doses to women with anovulatory infertility and strict criteria employed before the administration of hCG as the ovulatory trigger.

## SURGICAL OVULATION INDUCTION

Laparoscopic ovarian surgery has replaced ovarian wedge resection as the surgical treatment for clomiphene resistance in women with PCOS. It is free of the risks of multiple pregnancy and ovarian hyperstimulation and does not require intensive ultrasound monitoring. Furthermore, ovarian diathermy appears to be as effective as routine gonadotrophin therapy in the treatment of clomiphene-insensitive PCOS.[11–13] In addition, laparoscopic ovarian surgery is a useful therapy for anovulatory women with PCOS who fail to respond to clomiphene and need a laparoscopic assessment of their pelvis or in those living too far away from the hospital to attend for the intensive monitoring required for gonadotrophin therapy. Laparoscopic ovarian surgery reduces serum LH concentrations and is recommended for patients who persistently hypersecrete LH (see below). Surgery carries risks and should be performed by properly trained laparoscopic surgeons.

Wedge resection of the ovaries was initially described in 1935 by Stein and Leventhal[14] at the time when polycystic ovaries were diagnosed during a laparotomy. Ovarian biopsies taken to make the diagnosis were followed by ovulation. The rationale was to 'normalise' ovarian size and hence the endocrinopathy by removing between 50–75% of each ovary. A large review of 187 reports summarised data on 1079 ovarian wedge resections, with an overall ovulation rate of 80% and pregnancy of 62.5% (range, 13.5–89.5%).[15] Many years later, Donesky and Adashi[12] were able to increase the summated experience in the literature to 1766 treatments, with an average pregnancy rate of 58.8%. Wedge resection went out of favour in the 1970s when significant postoperative adhesion formation was recognised and the initial favourable pregnancy rates were not sustained.

Laparoscopic surgery has several obvious advantages over laparotomy and was first reported by Palmer[16] some years after the invention of his ovarian biopsy forceps. The initial reports were of multiple biopsies with cautery only to stop bleeding. Commonly employed methods for laparoscopic surgery include monopolar electrocautery (diathermy)[17] and laser[18] but multiple biopsy alone is less commonly used. In the first reported series, ovarian diathermy resulted in ovulation in 90% and conception in 70% of the 62 women treated.[17] The outcome of 62 pregnancies was no different from the normal population[19] and the miscarriage rate was 15%.

A number of subsequent studies produced similarly encouraging results, although the techniques used and degree of ovarian damage vary considerably. Gjonnaess[17] cauterized each ovary at 5–8 points, for 5–6 s at each point with 300–400 W. Using the same technique as Gjonnaess, Dabirashrafi and colleagues[20] reported mild to moderate adhesion formation in 20% of patients. Naether and colleagues[21] treated 5–20 points per ovary, with 400 W for approximately 1 s. They found that the rate of adhesions was 19.3% and that this was reduced to 16.6% by peritoneal lavage with saline.[22] In an earlier study, Naether and coworkers[23] found that the post-diathermy fall in serum testosterone concentration was proportional to the degree of ovarian damage, with up to 40 cauterisation sites being used in some patients. The greater the amount of damage to the surface of the ovary, the greater the risk of peri-ovarian adhesion formation. This lead Armar to develop a strategy of minimising the number of diathermy points.[24] We have employed Armar's technique, in which the ovary is simply cauterized at 4 points. We have not performed routine follow-up laparoscopy on our patients, but the high pregnancy rate (86% of those with no other pelvic abnormality) reported by Armar and Lachelin[25] indicates that the smaller number of diathermy points used leads to a low rate of significant adhesion formation.

The risk of peri-ovarian adhesion formation may be reduced by abdominal lavage and early second-look laparoscopy, with adhesiolysis if necessary.[26] Others have also used liberal peritoneal lavage to good effect.[24,27]. Greenblatt and Casper[28] found no correlation between the degree of ovarian damage and subsequent adhesion formation, and found no benefit from the adhesion barrier Interceed (Ethicon Ltd), as assessed by second look laparoscopy. In another interesting study, 40 women undergoing laser photocoagulation of the ovaries using an Nd-YAG laser set at 50 W at 20–25 points per ovary were randomised to a second-look laparoscopy and adhesiolysis.[29] Of those who underwent a second-look laparoscopy, adhesions described as minimal or mild were found in 68%; adhesiolysis did not appear to be necessary, as the cumulative conception rate after 6 months was 47% compared with 55% in the expectantly-managed group (not significant).

The difficulty with laparoscopic ovarian diathermy (LOD) is not knowing the 'dose response' for a particular patient. Our results show that LOD using 40 W for 4 s in 4 places on one ovary can lead to bilateral ovarian activity and ovulation (our usual protocol involves the same on each ovary);[27] our ovulation rate was 50% and conception rate 40% (some patients were sensitised to exogenous stimulation). It has been proposed that the degree of ovarian destruction should be determined by the size of the ovary.[30] Naether and colleagues reported their method of laparoscopic electrocautery of the ovarian surface (LEOS) which causes greater destruction of the ovary than the method we use, as they apply 400 W at 5–20 sites on each ovary.[30] Despite such a large amount of ovarian destruction, in Naether's series of 206 patients 45.2% of those who conceived required additional ovarian stimulation (with an 8% multiple pregnancy rate) and the overall miscarriage rate was 20%.[30] We may be dealing with different patient populations, as we recommend operation only for women with irregular, anovulatory cycles who have not responded to anti-oestrogen therapy; in Naether's series, approximately 24% of the women operated on had regular cycles and 15% were ovulating before their operation.

Unilateral ovarian diathermy may be insufficient to induce spontaneous ovulations and pregnancies in all patients and we would like to quantify better the 'dose' of diathermy that is required and evaluate how it should be adjusted for individual patients. We caution those practicing any form of ovarian destruction to strive to cause as little damage as is necessary in order to induce ovulation. In general, the correct dose of any therapy is the lowest that is effective. Furthermore, a combined approach may be suitable for some women whereby low dose diathermy is followed by low dose ovarian stimulation. Ostrzenski,[31] for example, commenced all his patients on either clomiphene or FSH therapy immediately after laser wedge resection and Farhi and colleagues[32] also demonstrated an increased ovarian sensitivity to gonadotrophin therapy after LOD.

An additional concern is the possibility of ovarian destruction leading to ovarian failure, an obvious disaster in a woman wishing to conceive. Cases of ovarian failure have been reported after both wedge resection and laparoscopic surgery.[13,33] An unfortunate vogue has developed whereby women with polycystic ovaries who have over-responded to **superovulation** for IVF are subjected to ovarian diathermy as the way of reducing the likelihood of subsequent OHSS.[34] If appropriately performed ovarian diathermy works by sensitising the ovary to FSH and ovarian diathermy certainly makes the clomiphene-resistant polycystic ovary sensitive to clomiphene,[32] then one could extrapolate that ovarian diathermy prior to superovulation for IVF should make the ovary **more**, and not less, likely to overstimulate. The amount of ovarian destruction that is required to reduce the chance of overstimulation is, therefore, likely to be considerable and one should be very cautious before proceeding with such an approach because of concerns about permanent ovarian atrophy.

LOD appears to be as effective as routine gonadotrophin therapy in the treatment of clomiphene-insensitive PCOS.[11]. Abdel Gadir and coworkers[11] randomised prospectively 88 patients, who had failed to conceive after six CC cycles, to receiving either hMG, FSH or LOD. No differences were found in the rates of ovulation or pregnancy between the two groups, although those treated with LOD had fewer cycles with multiple follicular growth and a lower rate of miscarriage.[11] This is the only prospective randomised study to have attempted to compare the two therapies and further studies with larger numbers are required.

An unfortunate feature of the majority of the reports on wedge resection is the poor characterisation of the patients such that many appear to have been ovulating prior to treatment. This problem also features in many reports that describe laparoscopic treatment, so that it is unclear whether patients are anovulatory prior to treatment, let alone whether they have polycystic ovaries in all cases. Laser treatment seems to be as efficacious as diathermy and may result in less adhesion formation;[35–37] the only study to compare the two techniques was non-randomised and reported similar ovulation and pregnancy rates but did not examine adhesion formation.[38] Various types of laser have been used from the $CO_2$ laser, to the Nd:YAG and KTP lasers. As with the use of laser in other spheres of laparoscopic surgery, whether laser or diathermy is employed appears to depend upon the preference of the surgeon and the availability of the equipment. A recent retrospective analysis of 118 cases of laparoscopic ovarian surgery reported a 12 month cumulative conception rate of 54%.[39] Those who had a shorter duration of infertility (of less than 3 years), had a higher pre-treatment LH concentration (>10 IU/l) and received diathermy rather than laser had a cumulative conception rate of 79%.[39]

## LAPAROSCOPIC OVARIAN SURGERY AND ENDOCRINE CHANGES

Whatever the mechanism of action of laparoscopic ovarian surgery, there is no doubt that, with restoration of ovarian activity, serum concentrations of LH and testosterone fall. The endocrine changes following ovarian diathermy have been explored in detail by a number of groups. Greenblatt and Casper[40] studied 6 patients and found that serum androgen concentrations fell to a nadir by the third postoperative day and this preceded a fall in serum oestradiol and LH concentrations, which then co-incided with a rise in serum FSH concentration by day 2–3. It was postulated that ovarian trauma impaired local production of androgens and hence a reduction in extra-ovarian production of oestrone, which in turn would decrease positive feedback on LH secretion. Negative feedback on FSH secretion would diminish concurrently, caused by both a decrease in peripheral oestrogens and also, possibly, ovarian inhibin.[40] Abdel Gadir and colleagues[41] found a significant fall in serum LH and testosterone concentrations and examined LH pulse frequency, which was unaltered following LOD. In a study of 11 patients treated by laser to the ovary, Rossmanith and coworkers[42] also noted no change in pulse frequency of LH secretion and observed an attenuation in GnRH-stimulated LH following treatment, suggesting an alteration of ovarian-pituitary feedback that affects the sensitivity of the pituitary to GnRH.

In two small series, ovulation was induced in approximately 70% of patients and the serum testosterone concentrations fell significantly, but no change was found in the mean serum LH concentrations.[43,44] Naether and colleagues[45] observed a decline in serum androgen concentrations and a slight increase in serum gonadotrophin levels. Most series, however, report a fall in both androgen and LH concentrations and an increase in FSH concentrations.[24,42] A fall in serum LH concentrations both increases the chance of conception and reduces the risk of miscarriage, as demonstrated by Armar and Lachelin,[25] who observed a miscarriage rate of 14% in 58 pregnancies compared with the expected miscarriage rate of 30–40% seen in reports of hormonal induction of ovulation in women with PCOS.

Whether patients respond to LOD appears to depend on their pre-treatment characteristics, with patients with high basal LH concentrations having a better clinical and endocrine outcome.[46] That study found that the pre-treatment testosterone level, body mass index and ovarian volume could not be used to predict outcome. We performed a small prospective randomised study in which women received either unilateral or bilateral LOD.[47] Unilateral diathermy restored bilateral ovarian activity, with the contralateral, untreated ovary often being the first to ovulate after the diathermy treatment. We also found that the only significant difference between the responders and non-responders was a post-diathermy fall in serum LH concentration.

The mechanism of ovulation induction by LOD is uncertain and the minimal damage to an unresponsive ovary either restores an ovulatory cycle or increases the sensitivity of the ovary to exogenous stimulation. Furthermore, the finding of an attenuated response of LH secretion to stimulation with GnRH[42] suggests an affect on ovarian–pituitary feedback and hence pituitary sensitivity to GnRH. Our study goes one step further by demonstrating that unilateral diathermy leads to bilateral ovarian activity, suggesting that ovarian diathermy may correct a perturbation of ovarian–pituitary feedback.[47] We suggest that the response of the ovary to injury leads to a local cascade of growth factors and those such as IGF-1, which interact with FSH, result in stimulation of follicular growth and the production of the hormone gonadotrophin surge attenuating/inhibitory factor (GnSAF/GnSIF) which leads to a fall in serum LH concentrations.[48]

## MEDICAL OR SURGICAL OVULATION INDUCTION?

Compared with medical ovulation induction, the additional advantages of laparoscopic diathermy are that it is performed once, intensive monitoring is not required, and multiple ovulation or ovarian hyperstimulation do not occur. Furthermore, only minimal ovarian damage is required to achieve this effect. The correct dose of diathermy to stimulate reliably the resumption of ovulatory cycles remains uncertain and the degree of permanent damage done to the ovary.

One of the strong arguments for the use of LOD as a therapy is the avoidance of multiple pregnancy. The risks of multiple pregnancy are significant with greater monitoring of the pregnancy required, problems with prenatal screening (particularly if there is discordancy for abnormality), increased incidence of pregnancy-induced hypertension, antepartum haemorrhage, preterm labour and surgical delivery. Neonatal mortality is 7 times higher in twins than singletons and 20 times higher in triplets and higher order births, while survivors have an increased risk of cerebral palsy and other neurological impairments. Furthermore, multiple pregnancies that occur in subfertile women appear to fare worse than those in otherwise normal women. Even if all children are born healthy, the parenting problems and stresses to the family unit are immense.

The possible association between epithelial ovarian cancer and ovulation induction therapies has been widely discussed following a retrospective case-controlled study from the US;[49] this did not provide adequate information about the drugs used and concerned a small number of cases of different histological types. Infertility is associated with an increased risk of ovarian cancer and suppression of ovarian activity (oral contraceptive use, pregnancy, etc.) reduces the risk. We have recently reviewed the literature on the association between ovulation induction and ovarian cancer and conclude, along with others, that more prospective data collection is required.[50] Whether laparoscopic ovarian surgery causes epithelial damage sufficient to increase the long-term risk of ovarian cancer is unknown.

Unifollicular ovulation induction requires a subtle approach, particularly in women with the PCOS. Gonadotrophin therapy adds appreciably to the cost of the treatment in assisted reproduction. The potential financial costs of a multiple pregnancy, particularly the neonatal intensive care facilities, are considerable. Other costs have to be counted in terms of the successful outcome of treatment with a low rate of miscarriage and the birth of healthy, preferably singleton, babies, with no health risks to their mothers. Laparoscopy ovarian surgery appears to provide a significant advantage: a single treatment that results in unifollicular ovulation, with correction of the endocrinopathy and an apparent low rate of miscarriage. Women usually

## Key points for clinical practice

- Laparoscopic ovarian surgery achieves rates of ovulation of 70–80% in women with clomiphene-resistant polycystic ovary syndrome.

- Clomiphene citrate remains first line therapy for ovulation induction in polycystic ovary syndrome.

- Obese patients with polycystic ovary syndrome should be encouraged to lose weight (BMI < 30 kg/m$^2$) before fertility treatment.

- Gonadotrophin therapy and laparoscopic ovarian diathermy are equally effective for clomiphene-resistant patients.

- Laparoscopic surgery should be performed by appropriately trained surgeons.

- The minimum amount of ovarian damage should be caused.

- Diathermy is recommended at 4 points on each ovary.

- An appropriate amount of ovarian damage will sensitise the ovary to FSH, whether endogenous or exogenous.

- Laparoscopic ovarian surgery requires less monitoring than gonadotrophin therapy and does not carry the risks of multiple pregnancy or ovarian hyperstimulation syndrome.

- Tubal patency may be assessed at the same time as laparoscopic ovarian surgery.

- The risks of laparoscopic ovarian surgery include the risks of an anaesthetic, peri-ovarian adhesions and ovarian destruction/failure.

require a test of tubal patency prior to gonadotrophin therapy and many would, therefore, have a laparoscopy. The main concern is the formation of adhesions and the potential for significant reduction in viable ovarian tissue, with the possibility of inducing premature ovarian failure. The evidence to date, however, is reassuring. The underlying principle of all methods of ovulation induction for women with polycystic ovary syndrome should be to use the lowest possible dose (of drug or surgery) to achieve unifollicular ovulation.

## References

1  Balen AH. The pathogenesis of the polycystic ovary syndrome. Lancet 1999; 354: 966–967
2  Balen AH, Conway GS, Kaltsas G et al. Polycystic ovary syndrome: the spectrum of the disorder in 1741 patients. Hum Reprod 1995; 10: 2705–2712
3  Dunaif A. Insulin resistance and the polycystic ovary syndrome: mechanisms and implication for pathogenesis. Endocr Rev 1997; 18: 774–800
4  Clark AM, Ledger W, Galletly C et al. Weight loss results in significant improvement in pregnancy and ovulation rates in anovulatory obese women. Hum Reprod 1995; 10: 2705–2712
5  Balen AH, Tan SL, Jacobs HS. Hypersecretion of luteinizing hormone: a significant cause of infertility and miscarriage. Br J Obstet Gynaecol 1993; 100: 1082–1089
6  Lockwood GM, Muttukrishna S, Groome NP, Matthews DR, Ledger WL. Mid-follicular phase pulses of inhibin B are absent in polycystic ovary syndrome and are initiated by successful laparoscopic ovarian diathermy: a possible mechanism for the emergence of the dominant follicle. J Clin Endocrinol Metab 1998; 83: 1730–1735
7  Hamilton-Fairley D, Kiddy D, Watson H, Paterson C, Franks S. Association of moderate obesity with poor pregnancy outcome in women with polycystic ovary syndrome treated with low dose gonadotrophins. Br J Obstet Gynaecol 1992; 99: 128–131
8  Kousta E, White DM, Franks S. Modern use of clomiphene citrate in induction of ovulation. Hum Reprod Update 1997; 3: 359–365
9  Balen AH, Braat DDM, West C, Patel A, Jacobs HS. Cumulative conception and live birth rates after the treatment of anovulatory infertility. An analysis of the safety and efficacy of ovulation induction in 200 patients. Hum Reprod 1994; 9: 1563–1570
10 Levene MI, Wild J, Steer P. Higher multiple births and the modern management of infertility in Britain. Br J Obstet Gynaecol 1992; 99: 607–613
11 Abdel Gadir A, Mowafi RS, Alnaser HMI, Alrashid AH, Alonezi OM, Shaw RW. Ovarian electrocautery versus human menopausal gonadotrophins and pure follicle stimulating hormone therapy in the treatment of patients with polycystic ovarian disease. Clin Endocrinol 1990; 33: 585–592
12 Donesky BW, Adashi EY. Surgically induced ovulation in the polycystic ovary syndrome: wedge resection revisited in the age of laparoscopy. Fertil Steril 1995; 63: 439–463
13 Cohen BM. Laser laparoscopy for polycystic ovaries. Fertil Steril 1989; 52: 167–168
14 Stein IF, Leventhal ML. Amenorrhoea associated with bilateral polycystic ovaries. Am J Obstet Gynecol 1935; 29: 181–191
15 Goldzieher JW, Axelrod LR. Clinical and biochemical features of polycystic ovarian disease. Fertil Steril 1963; 14: 631–653
16 Palmer R, de Brux J. Resultants histologiques, biochemiques et therapeutiques obtenus chez les femmes dont les ovaires avaient ete diagnostiques Stein-Leventhal a la coelioscopie. Bull Fed Soc Gynaecol Obstet Lang Fr 1967; 19: 405–412
17 Gjoannaess H. Polycystic ovarian syndrome treated by ovarian electrocautery through the laparoscope. Fertil Steril 1984; 41: 20–25
18 Daniell JF, Miller N. Polycystic ovaries treated by laparoscopic laser vaporization. Fertil Steril 1989; 51: 232–236
19 Gjoannaess H. The course and outcome of pregnancy after ovarian electrocautery with PCOS: the influence of body weight. Br J Obstet Gynaecol 1989; 96: 714–719

20 Dabirashrafi H, Mohamad K, Behjatnia Y *et al*. Adhesion formation after ovarian electrocauterization on patients with PCO syndrome. Fertil Steril 1991; 55: 1200–1201

21 Naether OGJ, Fischer R, Weise HC, Geiger-Kotzler L, Delfs T, Rudolf K. Laparoscopic electrocoagulation of the ovarian surface in infertile patients with polycystic ovarian disease. Fertil Steril 1993; 60: 88–94

22 Naether OGJ, Fischer R. Adhesion formation after laparoscopic electrocoagulation of the ovarian surface in polycystic ovary patients. Fertil Steril 1993; 60: 95–99

23 Naether OGJ, Weise HC, Fischer R. Treatment with electrocautery in sterility patients with polycystic ovarian disease. Geburtsh Frauenheilk 1991; 51: 920–924

24 Armar NA, McGarrigle HHG, Honour JW, Holownia P, Jacobs HS, Lachelin GCL. Laparoscopic ovarian diathermy in the management of anovulatory infertility in women with polycystic ovaries: endocrine changes and clinical outcome. Fertil Steril 1990; 53: 45–49

25 Armar NA, Lachelin GCL. Laparoscopic ovarian diathermy: an effective treatment for anti-oestrogen resistant anovulatory infertility in women with polycystic ovaries. Br J Obstet Gynaecol 1993; 100: 161–164

26 Naether OGJ. Significant reduction in adnexal adhesions following laparoscopic electrocautery of the ovarian surface by lavage and artificial ascites. Gynaecol Endosc 1995; 4: 17–19

27 Balen AH, Jacobs HS. Ovulation induction. In: Balen AH, Jacobs HS. (eds) Infertility in Practice. Edinburgh: Churchill Livingstone, 1997; 131–180

28 Greenblatt E, Casper RF. Adhesion formation after laparoscopic ovarian cautery for PCOS: lack of correlation with pregnancy rate. Fertil Steril 1993; 60: 766–769

29 Gurgan T, Urman B *et al*. The effect of short internal laparoscopic lysis of adhesions in pregnancy rates following Nd:YAG laser photocoagulation of PCOS. Obstet Gynecol 1992; 80: 45–47

30 Naether OGJ, Baukloh V, Fischer R, Kowalczyk T. Long-term follow-up in 206 infertility patients with polycystic ovarian syndrome after laparoscopic electrocautery of the ovarian surface. Hum Reprod 1994; 9: 2342–2349

31 Ostrzenski A. Endoscopic carbon dioxide laser ovarian wedge resection in resistant polycystic ovarian disease. Int J Fertil 1992; 37: 295–299

32 Farhi J, Soule S, Jacobs H. Effect of laparoscopic ovarian electrocautery on ovarian response and outcome of treatment with gonadotrophins in clomiphene citrate resistant patients with PCOS. Fertil Steril 1995; 64: 930–935

33 Toaff R, Toaff ME, Peyser MR. Infertility following wedge resection of the ovaries. Am J Obstet Gynecol 1976; 124: 92–96

34 Rimmington MR, Walker SM, Shaw RW. The use of laparoscopic ovarian electrocautery in preventing cancellation of in-vitro fertilization treatment cycles due to risk of ovarian hyperstimulation syndrome in women with polycystic ovaries. Hum Reprod 1997; 7: 1443–1447

35 Huber J, Hosmann J, Spona J. Polycystic ovarian syndrome treated by laser through the laparoscope. Lancet 1988; ii: 215

36 Daniell JF, Miller N. Polycystic ovaries treated by laparoscopic laser vaporization. Fertil Steril 1989; 51: 232–236

37 Keckstein G, Rossmanith W, Spatzier K, Schneider V, Borchers K, Steiner R. The effect of laparoscopic treatment of polycystic ovarian disease by $CO_2$-laser or Nd:YAG laser. Surg Endosc 1990; 4: 103–107

38 Heylen SM, Puttemans PJ, Brosens LH. Polycystic ovarian disease treated by laparoscopic argon laser capsule drilling: comparison of vaporization versus perforation technique. Hum Reprod 1994; 9: 1038–1042

39 Li TC, Saravelos H, Chow MS, Chisabingo R, Cooke ID. Factors affecting the outcome of laparoscopic ovarian drilling for polycystic ovary syndrome in women with anovulatory infertility. Br J Obstet Gynaecol 1998; 105: 338–344

40 Greenblatt E, Casper RF. Endocrine changes after laparoscopic ovarian cautery in polycystic ovarian syndrome. Am J Obstet Gynecol 1987; 42: 517–518

41 Abdel Gadir A, Khatim MS, Mowafi RS, Alnaser HMI, Alzaid HGN, Shaw RW. Hormonal changes in patients with polycystic ovarian disease after ovarian electrocautery or pituitary desensitization. Clin Endocrinol 1990; 32: 749–754

42 Rossmanith WG, Keckstein J, Spatzier K, Lauritzen C. The impact of ovarian laser surgery on the gonadotrophin secretion in women with polycystic ovarian disease. Clin Endocrinol 1991; 34: 223–230

43 Van der Weiden RMF, Alberda AT, de Jong FH, Brandenburg H. Endocrine effects of laparoscopic ovarian electrocautery in patients with polycystic ovarian disease, resistant to clomiphene citrate. Eur J Obstet Gynecol Reprod Biol 1989; 32: 157–162

44 Kovaks G, Buckler H, Bangah M *et al*. Treatment of anovulation due to PCOS by laparoscopic ovarian electrocautery. Br J Obstet Gynaecol 1991; 98: 30–35

45 Naether OGJ, Fischer R, Weise HC, Geiger-Kotzler L, Delfs T, Rudolf K. Laparoscopic electrocoagulation of the ovarian surface in infertile patients with polycystic ovarian disease. Fertil Steril 1993; 60: 88–94

46 Abdel Gadir A, Alnaser HMI, Mowafi RS, Shaw RW. The response of patients with polycystic ovarian disease to human menopausal gonadotrophin therapy after ovarian electrocautery or a luteinizing hormone-releasing hormone agonist. Fertil Steril 1992; 57: 309–313

47 Balen AH, Jacobs HS. A prospective study comparing unilateral and bilateral laparoscopic ovarian diathermy in women with the polycystic ovary syndrome. Fertil Steril 1994; 62: 921–925

48 Balen AH, Jacobs HS. Gonadotrophin surge attenuating factor – a missing link in the control of LH secretion? Clin Endocrinol 1991; 35: 399–402

49 Whittemore AS, Harris R, Itnyre J, and the Collaborative Ovarian Cancer Group. Characteristics relating to ovarian cancer risk: collaborative analysis of 12 US case-control studies. II Invasive epithelial ovarian cancers in white women. Am J Epidemiol 1992; 136: 1184–1203

50 Nugent D, Salha O, Balen AH, Rutherford AJ. Ovarian neoplasia and subfertility treatments. Br J Obstet Gynaecol 1998; 105: 584–591

Laparoscopic treatment of polycystic ovary syndrome

*Richard Kennedy*

# Aetiology, prevention and treatment of ovarian hyperstimulation syndrome

Ovarian hyperstimulation syndrome (OHSS) is an uncommon, but potentially life threatening, complication of ovarian stimulation by ovulation induction agents. This iatrogenic condition was first described following the use of gonadotrophins[1] used in ovulation induction, but is now most commonly seen following the use of super-ovulation regimens that are routinely used in assisted conception. The importance of the condition is two-fold. Firstly, with judicious management, its incidence and severity can be largely reduced. Secondly, as these cases are often admitted to a general gynaecology ward, it is important that all obstetricians and gynaecologists have a working knowledge of the principles of its pathogenesis and management.

The reported incidence of OHSS varies according to the study population. Ovarian hyperstimulation syndrome has rarely been reported to occur spontaneously,[2] although Meig's syndrome, a condition characterised by ascites and hydrothorax in association with a benign ovarian tumour, has similar features. The condition is very occasionally seen following the use of clomiphene citrate for ovulation induction in anovulatory infertility.[3] OHSS is unlikely to occur when gonadotrophins are used in a low dose regimen for ovulation induction.[4] Assisted conception techniques, such as in vitro fertilisation (IVF), normally require the intentional development of several follicles simultaneously (superovulation) and mild OHSS is relatively common in this situation. The reported incidence of severe OHSS in in vitro fertilization programmes varies between 0.5–10% and depends on a number of factors including the diagnostic classification used.[5,6] In our own series of 1734 stimulated IVF cycles between 1995–1998, the incidence of severe OHSS as judged by a haematocrit of greater than 0.45 and clinically significant ascites was 1.84%. The incidence of moderate OHSS not requiring admission is of the order of 5–10% of all IVF cycles.

**Mr Richard Kennedy** FRCOG, Consultant Obstetrician and Gynaecologist and Honorary Senior Lecturer, Centre for Reproductive Medicine, Walsgrave Hospitals NHS Trust, Clifford Bridge Road, Coventry CV2 2DX, UK

## PATHOGENESIS

Ovarian hyperstimulation syndrome is characterised by an increase in vascular permeability leading to a fluid shift from the intravascular to the extravascular space. This leads to reduced circulating volume, depletion of albumin and electrolytes and third space accumulation of fluid manifest by ascites and, rarely, hydrothorax.

The precise aetiology of OHSS is not known, although the condition is most often seen in cases where there has been multiple ovarian follicular development. The trigger for OHSS is the endogenous LH surge during a conventional ovulation induction cycle or exogenous human chorionic gonadotrophin (hCG) given during an IVF cycle, although cases have been described without luteinisation of the follicles.

The primary event in the development of OHSS is changing vascular permeability and theories for the causation have developed round the factor or factors which may be implicated in this event. A number of candidates have been proposed (Table 10.1).

High circulating levels of oestradiol are associated with an increased risk of OHSS and are often used as a predictor. However, the condition can occur in women with 17,20-desmolase deficiency who have low oestradiol.[7] Evidence from animal studies has shown that high dose oestradiol administered to rabbits does not induce OHSS. Furthermore, rabbits whose ovaries had been extra-peritonealized, were still capable of developing this condition.[8] Prostaglandin is known to be an active mediator in the inflammatory response and to effect vascular permeability. However, the use of prostaglandin synthetase inhibitors do not effect the outcome of OHSS and prostaglandins are unlikely to be the causative agent.[16] Peripheral levels of histamine have not been shown to rise in OHSS[17] and anti-histamines are not useful in its management.[18] Prolactin is an unlikely candidate, as anti-dopaminergic drugs have not been shown to reduce the incidence of OHSS in the rabbit model.[8] The renin–angiotensin mechanism is a possible factor[9] as evidenced by correlation of pro-renin levels with the LH peak,[10,11] raised plasma renin levels which correlate with the severity of OHSS[12,13] and the fact that angiotensin II enhances vascular permeability.[14,15]

Cytokines are key components of the inflammatory response, and their role in the pathogenesis of OHSS has been considered as they are known to alter vascular permeability. Evidence in support of this comes from experiments

**Table 10.1** Candidate factors for causation of OHSS

Oestrogen
Renin–angiotensin system
Prostaglandins
Histamine
Prolactin
Cytokines
Vascular endothelial growth factor (VEGF)
Interleukins (IL-2, IL-6, IL-8)

which have shown high levels of cytokines in ascitic fluid in patients with OHSS,[19] inhibition of vascular permeability in the rat model using a bradykinin-2 receptor antagonist,[20] inhibition of ascites formation in humans by Trasylol (which inhibits bradykinin synthesis) and increase in ascites formation by catopril (kininase II inhibitor).[21,22] Similarly, members of the interleukin family, particularly IL-1, IL-6 and IL-8, have also been shown to be implicated in the mediation of vascular permeability and have high levels in ascitic fluid taken from patients with OHSS.[23,24]

Vascular endothelial growth factor (VEGF) is currently the leading contender as primary mediator of vascular permeability changes in OHSS.[25] This view is supported by its properties as a potent mitogen of macrophages, chemo-attractant of endothelial cells and mediator of vascular permeability. Messenger RNA expression of VEGF is maximal in late follicular phase granulosa and theca cells.[26] Messenger RNA expression of VEGF is also induced by the mid-cycle LH surge.[27] Further evidence comes from the fact that ovarian follicular levels of VEGF found in in vitro fertilisation are much higher than serum levels[28] and antisera to VEGF reduces vascular permeability.[25]

A change in vascular permeability appears to be the primary event in OHSS, but unanswered questions remain, as ascites may have an extra-ovarian origin[29] and the precise role of VEGF and other possible mediators remain to be clarified.[30] Two main theories are currently expounded.

## PERIPHERAL ARTERIOLAR VASODILATATION

Balasch and colleagues[31] presented evidence to support peripheral arteriolar vasodilatation as the primary event in the pathogenesis of OHSS. They argue that the haemodynamic effects are similar to the pregnant state and that vasodilatation is likely to be mediated by increased levels of oestradiol which are normally elevated in this condition. The homeostatic response to this vascular change occurs through baroreceptors within the renal tubular juxta-glomerular apparatus causing activation of the renin–angiotensin–aldosterone system and sympathetic nervous system. In addition, anti-diuretic hormone

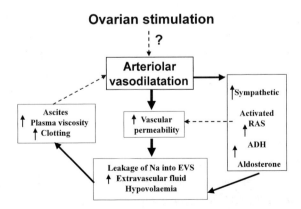

**Fig. 10.1** Decreased circulating volume in the pathogenesis of ovarian hyperstimulation syndrome.

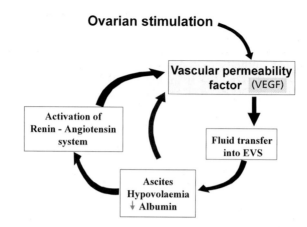

**Ovarian stimulation**

**Vascular permeability factor** (VEGF)

**Activation of Renin - Angiotensin system**

**Fluid transfer into EVS**

**Ascites Hypovolaemia ↓ Albumin**

**Fig. 10.2** The role of VEGF in the pathogenesis of ovarian hyperstimulation syndrome

(ADH) is released. These compensatory mechanisms act by retaining sodium which contribute to the fluid shift to the extravascular space (Fig. 10.1).

## INCREASED CAPILLARY PERMEABILITY

This theory is supported by many authors who have proposed substance(s) released from the ovarian follicles that mediate the increase in vascular permeability characteristic of OHSS. This causes a fluid shift to the extravascular space which, in turn, lowers peripheral circulating volume and arteriolor filling. This, in turn, triggers the renin–angiotensin–aldosterone (RAS) system as a secondary homeostatic mechanism. The RAS system further aggravates the condition by increasing fluid and sodium retention (Fig. 10.2).

## CLINICAL PRESENTATION AND CLASSIFICATION

Patients almost always give a history of exposure to ovulation induction agents although very rare cases have been reported of this condition arising spontaneously.[32] The drug regimen most likely to result in OHSS is pituitary densitization with luteinizing hormone releasing hormone analogues (LHRHa) followed by stimulation with urinary-derived human menopausal gonadotrophins or recombinant follicle stimulating hormone. This is the standard stimulation protocol used for IVF in the UK. Its purpose is to suppress the spontaneous release of LH allowing control of the timing of oocyte recovery. Exogenous hCG is given in the late follicular phase to cause luteinization of the follicles prior to oocyte retrieval. If hCG is not given, OHSS is highly unlikely. If LHRH analogues are not used, OHSS can result through the spontaneous release of LH, although the incidence is reduced.

The characteristic features are related to third space accumulation which presents as abdominal distension leading to discomfort and respiratory difficulties. Hydrothorax may occur in the most severe cases and this further compromises respiration. The high circulating levels of oestradiol may cause

**Table 10.2** Clinical classification of ovarian hyperstimulation syndrome

|  | Ovary | Clinical | Blood |
|---|---|---|---|
| Mild | 5–10 cm | Abdominal distension ± GI upset Normal renal function | Haematocrit < 0.45 WBC <15,000 |
| Moderate | > 10 cm | Moderate ascites | Haematocrit < 0.45 WBC < 15,000 Normal renal function |
| Severe | > 12 mm | Marked ascites Abdominal distension Dyspneoa Hypovolaemia | Haematocrit > 0.45 WBC > 15,999 Renal function deteriorating |

nausea and this, together with the depleted intravascular volume, leads to diminished urinary output. Ultimately, if untreated, the hypovolaemia leads to renal impairment. The patient is in a hypercoagulable state as a consequence of several factors and may rarely present with venous thrombosis. Finally, because OHSS occurs most frequently in cases where there has been excessive ovarian response to stimulation, the ovaries will be markedly enlarged, usually greater than 10 cm in diameter. In these cases, the enlarged ovaries are easily palpable in the lower abdomen and, if the empty follicles have filled with blood, will be painful and tender.

## CLASSIFICATION OF OVARIAN HYPERSTIMULATION SYNDROME

Various classifications for OHSS have been proposed[33,34] based on a variety of clinical, ultrasound, biochemical and haematological parameters (Table 10.2). These detailed classifications can be helpful in comparative studies; but, for practical purposes, a more simplified approach will help in management decisions. The major concern is to identify the patient at risk of developing severe OHSS who, with prompt admission and pro-active management, will follow a less serious course. The key parameters that guide this decision are shown in Table 10.3.

**Table 10.3** Simplified management classification of OHSS

**Patient to be admitted**

 Marked abdominal distension with ascites and/or haematocrit ≥0.45 and/or significant disturbance in fluid balance

**Observe as an out-patient**

 Minimal abdominal distension and haematocrit < 0.45 and normal fluid intake and output

## INDICATORS OF RISK

Several factors identify a women as being at increased risk of OHSS. The most important are the presence of polycystic ovaries (PCO) and a previous history of OHSS.[35,34] During an assisted conception cycle, a scan is carried out early in the follicular phase (baseline scan) which provides the opportunity to assess ovarian morphology. In cases of PCO or when the previous response to ovarian stimulation has been excessive, the strength of stimulation is modified to reduce the dosage of follicle stimulating hormone (FSH).

Laparoscopic ovarian diathermy has been advocated as a treatment for PCO related anovulatory infertility. A recent study[36] investigated the impact of this technique on the incidence of OHSS in women with polycystic ovaries undergoing IVF. A significantly decreased cycle cancellation rate due to excess ovarian response was found in the group receiving ovarian diathermy, but no difference in any other parameter.

Other factors increasing risk of OHSS are decreasing age and the drug regimen used for stimulation. The routine use of pituitary desensitisation with LHRH analogues has increased the risk of OHSS by prolonging and enhancing follicular recruitment.[37,38] The introduction of recombinant FSH for ovulation induction appears to make no difference to the incidence of OHSS,[39] but early experience with LHRH antagonists suggests that their use may be helpful in reducing risk.[40,41] In vitro maturation of immature oocytes recovered from unstimulated ovaries is a new technique being developed as a modification of IVF. This involves recovering oocytes early in the follicular phase from small ovarian follicles (less than 9 mm in diameter) which have been unexposed to exogenous FSH. The immature eggs are cultured in vitro for several days and fertilised prior to embryo transfer. This technique could potentially eliminate the need for gonadotrophin stimulation and thus the risk of OHSS.[42]

In the later stages of ovarian stimulation for IVF, two other parameters determine risk for developing OHSS, namely serum oestradiol and the number of developing ovarian follicles. Several studies have presented criteria for determining risk to provide guidance for clinical management.[43-46] However, because of the variation in oestradiol assay and the inter and intra-operator differences in assessment of ovarian stimulation,[47] centres providing IVF should develop their own criteria. In our own series of patients with severe OHSS, the mean oestradiol was 19,786 pmol/l and the mean number of follicles greater than 14 mm diameter was 17.4. As a guide, a serum oestradiol of greater than 15,000 pmol/l or the presence of greater than 20 ovarian follicles on the day of hCG injection, would place the women at increased risk and require consideration of preventative measures. More recently, Agarwal[48] has demonstrated that assay of vascular epidermal growth factor (VEGF) improves risk prediction of OHSS in IVF when combined with a number of parameters including oestradiol, number of follicles, number of oocytes recovered and percentage of patients with PCO. In this study, a likelihood ratio test based on logistic regression modelling using unit change in predictive criteria was used producing sensitivity, specificity and positive predictive

**Table 10.4** Possible measures to prevent ovarian hyperstimulation syndrome

| |
|---|
| Avoid hCG (treatment cancellation) |
| Delay hCG – 'coasting' |
| Reduce hCG dose |
| Surrogate hCG (LH agonist) |
| Prophylactic albumin |
| Aspirate all follicles |
| Cryopreservation (avoid pregnancy) |
| Elective embryo cryopreservation |
| Avoid hCG in luteal phase |

value (PPV) for each marker. When combined with number of follicles, presence of PCO and oestradiol level, the rise in VEGF had a 90% sensitivity and 93.8% specificity for moderate and severe OHSS with a PPV of 60.0%.

In the absence of biochemical markers or excessive follicular response on ultrasound, the unexpected recovery of large numbers of oocytes (greater than 20) will also place the patient at increased risk of OHSS.

## PREVENTION OF OHSS

The trigger for OHSS is hCG and the only certain way of preventing this syndrome is to withhold its administration and cancel the cycle. This is very upsetting for the couple and has significant financial implications. Unfortunately, using the aforementioned parameters, the accuracy of prediction is low[49] and many cycles cancelled on the basis of ultrasound and biochemical markers would be lost unnecessarily. Several measures have been advocated to reduce the possibility of OHSS in cases deemed to be at risk (Table 10.4). None of these will eliminate OHSS and none have been shown to be beneficial in the context of large prospective randomized controlled trials; nevertheless, until the sensitivity of risk identification is increased, their use should be considered in high risk cases.

### Reducing hCG stimulation and surrogate hCG
Human chorionic gonadotrophin is the trigger for OHSS and patients at risk should be given a reduced dose prior to oocyte recovery or ovulation. This may reduce the severity, but not the likelihood, of the condition. Another approach has been to use the agonist effect of gonadotrophin releasing hormone analogues (GnRHa) to trigger an endogenous LH surge, thus avoiding the need for exogenous hCG administration which has a much longer half-life. Lewit and colleagues demonstrated a complete avoidance of OHSS in their study using this technique,[50] but until further trials are undertaken it cannot be advocated in routine practice.

### 'Coasting' – delaying administration of hCG
This approach involves delaying the administration of hCG for several days after the ovarian follicles have reached maturity during which time the plasma

oestradiol levels fall. Sher[51] reported avoidance of severe complications, but not elimination of OHSS, in 17 at risk patients following prolonged coasting. Dhont and colleagues[52] carried out a case controlled study and demonstrated an odds ratio for OHSS in the 'coasted' group of 0.11 (95% CI, 0.01–0.86) with a significantly reduced egg yield, but no difference in pregnancy rate. The mean duration of 'coasting' in this study was 1.9 days. Waldenstrom and colleagues[53] carried out a multi-centre prospective non-randomised study to evaluate coasting in a group of markedly hyperstimulated women (greater than 25 large follicles) with a mean coasting interval of 4.3 days. They reported no cases of severe OHSS with a reduced egg yield, but a pregnancy rate of 42% per cycle. Delayed administration of hCG provides a reasonable compromise between cycle cancellation and risk of OHSS. The maximum 'window' for delay is not clear and all studies show a reduction in egg yield. The quality of oocytes recovered after delayed hCG is not apparently affected as judged by embryo quality and the maintenance of satisfactory pregnancy rates.

### Elective cryopreservation of embryos

The primary stimulus to OHSS is hCG and invariably the condition is more severe and its course more protracted when pregnancy results. This is due to the increased levels of endogenous hCG, arising from the developing syncytiotrophoblast which acts to perpetuate the process. The advent of successful embryo cryopreservation has led to the possibility of limiting the severity of OHSS by avoiding pregnancy whilst at the same time maintaining the possibility of a pregnancy resulting from the replacement of thawed embryos in a subsequent non-stimulated cycle. Several studies have demonstrated benefit from this technique, but while the severity and duration of OHSS is reduced the condition is not avoided and the pregnancy rates resulting from replacement of frozen embryos are generally lower.[44,54–56]

### Prophylactic albumin and substitutes

Asch and coworkers,[43] in a non-randomised study of patients at high risk, gave albumin at the time of oocyte recovery, before established OHSS had developed. They reported no cases of OHSS in the treatment group. Three small randomised controlled trials (RCT) have subsequently shown a significant reduction in the incidence of OHSS in 'at risk' patients given prophylactic albumin at the time of egg collection.[57–59] Shaker,[60] in a small RCT, compared albumin with elective cryopreservation and showed no difference in the incidence of OHSS. A number of case series and retrospective analyses have shown no benefit.[61–63] The pathogenesis of OHSS centres on increased vascular permeability and the role of various substances in promoting this event. The rationale for the use of prophylactic albumin is to act as a carrier protein to prevent leakage of vasoactive substances into the extravascular space. However, there are concerns about the use of albumin in this context. The relatively small size of the molecule allows it to pass more easily into the extravascular space and, in addition, there are the well known risks of viral transmission and anaphylaxis associated with human blood products.[64] Albumin substitutes have been proposed and hydroxyethyl starch[65] was investigated in a RCT and showed a significant reduction in mild and moderate OHSS, but no reduction in severe OHSS.

## Immunoglobulins

Abramov[66] has recently demonstrated significantly lower levels of IgG and IgA gammaglobulins in the plasma of patients with severe OHSS. In a study subjecting rabbits to gonadotrophin stimulation, Orvieto[67] reported prevention of severe OHSS in those given intravenous immunoglobulin. These results suggest that immunoglobulin therapy may have a future role in the management of OHSS.

## Luteal phase support

Patients undergoing in vitro fertilization following pituitary densitisation and gonadotrophin stimulation are normally given luteal phase support because of GnRH suppression of endogenous LH and corpus luteum function. Soliman and colleagues[68] carried out a meta-analysis of RCTs to evaluate the place of luteal phase support and found that pregnancy rates were higher with hCG compared to progesterone, but at the expense of a higher incidence of OHSS. Mochtar and colleagues[69] compared progesterone alone and in combination with hCG and found no difference in the pregnancy rate, but a higher incidence of OHSS in the hCG group. Progesterone is the most frequently used luteal phase support in the UK, the type of preparation having no bearing on the incidence of OHSS. The use of hCG in those cases with no risk factors is unlikely to increase the risk of OHSS significantly and may improve treatment outcome, but at the present time progesterone appears to be the luteal phase support of choice.

## TREATMENT OF ESTABLISHED OHSS AND ITS COMPLICATIONS

The management of established OHSS should be undertaken under the supervision of a specialist in reproductive medicine who is familiar with ovulation induction and superovulation regimens. In the event of a patient being admitted to a general gynaecology unit 'out of hours', the case should be discussed with the specialist responsible for the infertility management or a specialist at the local unit providing assisted conception services. Treatment is aimed at limiting the risk of serious and life threatening complications the most common of which are thrombo-embolic (Table 10.5).

## COMPLICATIONS

The reason for the increased tendency to thrombo-embolic problems is not clearly understood, but is likely to be multi-factorial. Several authors have

**Table 10.5** Complications of ovarian hyperstimulation syndrome

Thrombo-embolic
Renal failure
Ovarian tortion
Intra-abdominal bleeding
Gastrointestinal symptoms
Respiratory compromise and ARDS
Liver dysfunction

reported changes in coagulation factors during OHSS leading to a hypercoagulable state,[70–72] although this is not common to all patients. These changes may be related to the supraphysiological plasma levels of oestradiol; however, the most important factor is likely to be haemoconcentration resulting from the hypovolaemic state as manifest by a raised haematocrit. Other factors include ovarian enlargement leading to pressure on the pelvic veins and immobilisation. Although thrombo-embolism is a rare complication of OHSS, there seems to be a propensity for upper vein and cerebral vein thrombosis and, rarely, this may be the primary presentation.[73]

Other complications relate to the pathophysiological changes of hypo-volaemia and third space accumulation. Oliguria results from reduced renal blood flow as a result of hypovolaemia. If uncorrected, this will ultimately result in renal failure. Respiratory difficulties are initially due to abdominal distension with diaphragmatic splinting and hydrothorax, but adult respiratory distress syndrome (ARDS) may rarely result from increased vascular permeability in the pulmonary circulation. Gastrointestinal symptoms and liver dysfunction relate to the high serum levels of oestradiol and raised intra-abdominal pressure.

## TREATMENT

The principles of treatment are outlined in Table 10.6. The first decision is when to admit the patient to hospital (Table 10.2). Factors to consider are the degree of risk of OHSS, the accessibility of the patient to regular out-patient attendance, the degree of symptoms and whether prophylactic measures have been employed to avoid pregnancy (elective cryopreservation). If the case is to be managed as an out-patient, daily visits to the clinic may be necessary with estimations of haematocrit (HCT), white cell count (WBC), urea and electrolytes and liver function. A haematocrit greater than 0.44 or abnormal renal or liver function will indicate admission. Worsening abdominal distension, even with a normal HCT, will also require admission.

## INITIAL THERAPY

Following admission, early and effective correction of hypovolaemia is essential to improve renal perfusion and reverse the haemoconcentration. Hartmann's solution or normal saline, with added potassium if required, is first line therapy. The use of albumin to correct hypovolaemia and raise plasma oncotic pressure

**Table 10.6** Treatment of ovarian hyperstimulation syndrome

| |
|---|
| Close monitoring of 'at risk' patients |
| Low threshold for admission |
| Involve 'expert' help at an early stage |
| Correct hypovolaemia |
| Prophylactic heparin |
| Drainage of 3rd space fluid accumulation |
| Avoid surgical intervention |

is controversial. Recent concern has been expressed over the use of human albumin following a Cochrane meta-analysis of RCTs investigating the use of human albumin in the critically ill patient. The Cochrane review,[64] although not including cases of severe OHSS, suggests that this strategy may be detrimental because of the tendency of albumin to pass into the extravascular space, worsening the oncotic gradient and further aggravating the fluid shift out of the intravascular compartment. Taking death as the outcome measure, the relative risk (RR) to a patient with hypovolaemia or hypoalbuminaemia receiving albumin was 1.46 (95% CI, 0.97–2.22) and 1.69 (95% CI, 1.07–2.67, respectively. Further studies are required to resolve this issue. Artificial plasma expanders such as Haemaccel will give temporary relief only, but the use of hydroxyethyl starch has been recommended because of its larger molecular weight and longer half-life.[65]

Because of the risk of thrombo-embolic complications, heparin should be given in a prophylactic dose, although bleeding into the ovarian follicles may be aggravated. Mannitol or dopamine may be required in oliguric patients and analgesia should avoid the use of prostaglandin synthetase inhibitors because of their adverse effect on renal blood flow.[74]

## MONITORING

Urinary output and fluid balance should be monitored closely, together with blood pressure, temperature and respiratory rate. Daily abdominal girth measurements will give some indication of deteriorating ascites. Haematological and biochemical parameters are important indicators of disease progression and will help to manage fluid replacement. Initially, they should be carried out on a daily basis. An in-dwelling catheter may be needed if urinary output is poor or if there is vulval oedema causing voiding difficulties. Pulse oximetry is needed when there are respiratory problems or significant pleural effusions. Additional monitoring will depend on the severity of the condition but in the most severe cases transfer to an intensive care unit may be required.

## DRAINAGE OF THIRD SPACE ACCUMULATION

Drainage of abdominal fluid is a key step in the management. The decision to perform this procedure is determined by the degree and progression of abdominal distension and the effect this has on respiratory effort. When the abdomen is tense and ascites is evident both clinically and on ultrasound, early drainage of fluid will bring immediate relief not only to the abdominal discomfort and respiratory difficulties but also to the urinary output.[75] In addition, the ascitic fluid is rich in cytokines implicated in the alterations in vascular permeability and drainage should limit the course of the illness. Drainage is normally carried out by abdominal paracentesis which should be carried out under ultrasound guidance to avoid the ovaries which are normally large, vascular and easily damaged. Drainage through the Pouch of Douglas has also been described using the technique of ultrasound guided needle aspiration.[76] As much fluid as possible should be removed during the

Aetiology, prevention and treatment of ovarian hyperstimulation syndrome procedure and, providing the hypovolaemia has been corrected, continuous drainage has no risk. Long-term drainage is not recommended because of the risk of sepsis, although re-accumulation of ascites with the need for further drainage is sometimes required.

## SURGICAL TREATMENT

Surgical intervention is rarely required and best avoided. The ultrasound appearance of a multiple cystic ovary more than 10 cm in diameter, coupled with free fluid, abdominal distension and pain, may tempt a generalist into a laparotomy. However, the ovaries in OHSS are large, vascular and easily traumatised and inevitably return to normal with conservative management. Laparotomy should not be undertaken except in rare cases where tortion is suspected or if there is evidence of significant intraperitoneal bleeding. Co-incidental ectopic pregnancy or heterotopic pregnancy are also possibilities. This diagnosis should be clear with vaginal ultrasound and serial hCG titres, although interpretation of imaging is made more difficult due to the presence of large multi-cystic ovaries and free fluid in the pelvis due to the ascites. If surgery is contemplated, it should only be carried out by an experienced gynaecologist or specialist in reproductive medicine.

## PREGNANCY AND OHSS

Pregnancy rates are reported to be higher in those patients who develop OHSS following IVF-ET.[47,77] This is not surprising when the risk factors for this condition are also good prognostic indicators for outcome of IVF that is age and high egg yield. However, Aboulghar and colleagues, reported that fertilization rates were reduced in patients with OHSS, although embryo quality and pregnancy rates were not affected.[78] Ovarian hyperstimulation syndrome runs a more severe and protracted course when pregnancy results due to the secretion of hCG by the very early feto-placental unit compounding the process. Abramov and colleagues have recently reported the obstetric outcome of a large series of cases from Israel where early pregnancy was complicated by severe OHSS. In this study, they found a significantly higher rate of miscarriage, low birth weight and preterm delivery in both singleton and multiple pregnancies, although other confounding factors such as age were not taken into account.[79] These observed changes may relate to poorer oocyte quality in patients with polycystic ovaries or the environment of the peri-implantation embryo.

## CONCLUSIONS

The use of gonadotrophins for follicular stimulation has risen sharply with the increasing use of assisted conception techniques. Approximately 30,000 IVF cycles are carried out in the UK each year, and an unknown number of other assisted conception treatments with ovulation induction cycles requiring gonadotrophin stimulation. Ovarian hyperstimulation syndrome is an iatrogenic complication of such treatment and may occur in up to 10% of cases. Mild and moderate cases account for the majority, but rarely severe and life-threatening cases of OHSS can occur. Risk factors such as age, previous response and the presence of polycystic ovaries identify about 50% of the cases at risk. The strength of response to the stimulation regimen also predicts risk. Several strategies are possible to reduce the severity of the condition, but only avoidance of hCG will prevent its occurrence. Treatment must involve specialist help and the cornerstones are prompt correction of hypovolaemia and drainage of ascites. Figure 10.3 summarises in an algorithm the key aspects to the management of this disorder. Because of the unique aspects of this condition and its management, the adoption of local protocols by all acute gynaecology units is recommended based on Figure 10.3.

Aetiology, prevention and treatment of ovarian hyperstimulation syndrome

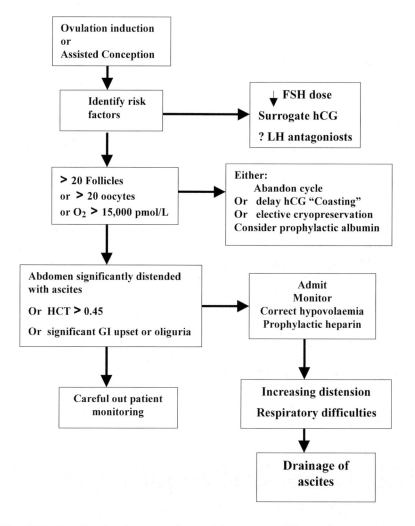

**Fig. 10.3** Algorithm for the prevention and management of ovarian hyperstimulation syndrome.

## Key points for clinical practice

- OHSS is an iatrogenic condition consequent upon the use of gonadotrophins used for ovulation induction and assisted conception.

- Polycystic ovaries are the main risk factor for the development of OHSS.

- All women receiving gonadotrophins require regular ultrasound monitoring to detect excessive follicular response which increases the risk of OHSS.

- The pathological basis of OHSS is increased vascular permeability.

- The clinical manifestations are due to a fluid shift from the intravascular to extravascular compartment leading to hypovolaemia, ascites and respiratory difficulties.

- OHSS only occurs once hCG has been given.

- Prevention includes the use of albumin, delayed hCG and elective cryopreservation of embryos, but will not eliminate the condition.

- Cases should be managed by a specialist in reproductive medicine.

- Haematocrit is a key marker of the severity of the condition.

- Management includes admission, fluid replacement and prophylactic heparin

- Early drainage of significant ascites under ultrasound guidance will aid resolution.

- Surgical intervention should be avoided unless indicated by additional pathology.

- The condition is self-limiting, but resolution is delayed by concomitant pregnancy.

## References

1  Mazer C, Ravetz E. Effect of combined administration of chorionic gonadotrophin and pituitary synergist on human ovary. Am J Obstet Gynecol 1941; 41: 474
2  Zalel Y, Katz Z, Caspi B *et al*. Spontaneous ovarian hyperstimulation syndrome concomitant with spontaneous pregnancy in a women with polycystic ovarian disease. Am J Obstet Gynecol 1992; 167: 122–124
3  Southan AL, Janovsky NA. Massive ovarian hyperstimulation with clomiphene citrate. JAMA 1962; 200: 443
4  Forman RG, Frydman R, Egan D. Severe ovarian hyperstimulation syndrome using agonists of gonadotrophin releasing hormone for in vitro fertilization: European series and proposal for prevention. Fertil Steril 1990; 53: 502–509
5  Hamilton-Fairley D, Kiddy D, Watson L *et al*. Low-dose gonadotrophin therapy for ovulation induction in 100 women with polycystic ovary syndrome. Hum Reprod 1991; 6: 1095–1099
6  MacDougall MJ, Tan SL, Jacobs HS. In-vitro fertilization and ovarian hyperstimulation syndrome. Hum Reprod 1992; 7: 579–600

7   Pride SM, James C, Ho Yuen BH. The ovarian hyperstimulation syndrome. Semin Reprod Endocrinol 1990; 8: 247–260

8   Meirow D, Schenker J, Rosler A. Ovarian hyperstimulation syndrome with low oestradiol in no-classical 17 alpha hydroxylase, 17-20 lyase deficiency: what is the role of oestrogens? Hum Reprod 1996; 11: 2119–2121

9   Ong ACM, Eisen V, Rennie DP, Homburg R, Lachelin GCL, Jacobs HS. Pathogenesis of ovarian hyperstimulation syndrome: a possible role for ovarian renin. Clin Endocrinol 1991; 34: 43–49

10  Sealey JE, Atlas SA, Gloriosi N et al. Cyclical secretion of prorenin during the menstrual cycle: synchronization with luteinizing hormone and progesterone. Proc Natl Acad Sci USA 1985; 82: 8705–8709

11  Sealey JE, Cholst I, Glorioso N et al. Sequential changes in plasma luteinizing hormone and plasma prorenin during the menstrual cycle. J Clin Endocrinol Metab 1987; 63: 1–5

12  Delbaere A, Bergmann PI, Gervy-Decoster C, Camu M, de Maertelaer V, Englert Y. Prorenin and active renin concentrations in plasma and ascites during severe ovarian hyperstimulation syndrome. Hum Reprod 1997; 12: 236–240

13  Navot D, Margalioth EJ, Laufer N et al. Direct correlation between plasma renin activity and severity of the ovarian hyperstimulation syndrome. Fertil Steril 1987; 48: 57–61

14  Delbaere A, Bergmann PJM, Gervy-Decoster C et al. Increased angiotensin II in ascites during severe ovarian hyperstimulation syndrome: role of pregnancy and ovarian gonadotrophin stimulation. Fertil Steril 1997; 67: 1038–1045

15  Berg PA, Navot D. Ovarian hyperstimulation syndrome: a review of pathophysiology. J Assist Reprod Genet 1992; 9: 429–438

16  Borenstein R, Elchalal U, Lunenfeld B, Shoham Schwartz Z. Severe ovarian hyperstimulation syndrome: a re-evaluated therapeutic approach. Fertil Steril 1989; 51: 791–795

17  Erlik Y, Naot Y, Friedman M. Histamine levels in ovarian hyperstimulation syndrome. Obstet Gynecol 1979; 53: 580

18  Gergely RZ, Paldi E, Erlik Y et al. Treatment of ovarian hyperstimulation syndrome by anti-histamine. Obstet Gynecol 1976; 47: 83–85

19  Revel A, Barak V, Lavy Y et al. Characterization of intraperitoneal cytokines and nitrites in women with severe ovarian hyperstimulation syndrome. Fertil Steril 1996; 66: 66–71

20  Ujioka T, Matsuura K, Tanaka N, Okamura H. Involvement of ovarian kini-kallikrein system in the pathophysiology of ovarian hyperstimulation syndrome: studies in a rat model. Hum Reprod 1998; 11: 3009–3015

21  Kobayashi H, Okada Y, Asahina T, Gotoh J, Terao T. The kallikrein-kinin system, but not vascular endothelial growth factor, plays a role in the increased vascular permeability associated with ovarian hyperstimulation syndrome. J Mol Endocrinol 1998; 20: 363–374

22  Simon C, Caballero-Campo P, Garcia-Velasco JA, Pellicer A. Potential implications of chemokines in reproductive function: an attractive idea. J Reprod Immunol 1998; 38: 169–193

23  Friedlander MA, de Mola JR, Goldfarb JM. Elevated levels of interleukin-6 in ascites and serum in women with ovarian hyperstimulation syndrome. Fertil Steril 1993; 60: 826–832

24  Mathur RS, Jenkins JM, Bansal AS. The possible role of the immune system in the aetiopathogenesis of ovarian hyperstimulation syndrome. Hum Reprod 1997; 12: 2629–2634

25  McClure N, Healy DL, Paw R et al. Vascular endothelial growth factor as a capillary permeability agent in ovarian hyperstimulation syndrome. Lancet 1994; 344: 235–243

26  Kamat BR, Brown LF, Manseau EJ, Senger DR, Dvorak HF. Expression of vascular endothelial growth factor by human granulosa and theca lutein cells. Role of corpus luteum development. Am J Pathol 1995; 146: 157–165

27  Neulen J, Zhaoping Y, Raczek S et al. Human chorionic gonadotrophin dependent expression of vascular endothelial growth factor in human granulosa cells and importance in ovarian hyperstimulation syndrome. J Clin Endocrinol Metab 1995; 80: 1967–1971

28  Lee A, Christenson LK, Stouffer RL, Bury KA, Patton PE. Vascular endothelial growth factor levels in serum and follicular fluid of patients undergoing in vitro fertilization. Fertil Steril 1997; 68: 305–311

68 Soliman S, Daya S, Collins J, Hughes EG. The role of luteal phase support in infertility treatment: a meta-analysis of randomized trials. Fertil Steril 1994; 6: 1068–1076

69 Mochtar MH, Hogerzeil HV, Mol BWJ. Progesterone alone versus progesterone combined with hCG as luteal support in GnRHa/HMG induced IVF cycles: a randomised clinical trial. Hum Reprod 1996; 11: 1602–1605

70 Aune B, Hoie KE, Oian P et al. Does ovarian stimulation for in vitro fertilization induce a hypercoagulable state? Hum Reprod 1991; 6: 925–927

71 Kodama H, Takeda S, Fukuda J et al. Activation of plasma kinin system correlated with severe coagulation disorders in patients with ovarian hyperstimulation syndrome. Hum Reprod 1997; 12: 891–895

72 Balasch J, Reverter JC, Fabregues F et al. Increased induced monocyte tissue factor expression by plasma from patients with severe ovarian hyperstimulation syndrome. Fertil Steril 1996; 66: 608–613

73 Stewart JA, Hamilton PJ, Murdoch AP. Thromboembolic disease associated with ovarian and assisted conception techniques. Hum Reprod 1997; 12: 2167–2173

74 Clive DM, Stoff JS. Renal syndromes associated with nonsteroidal anti-inflammatory drugs. N Engl J Med 1984; 310: 563–572

75 Abdalla HI, Rizk B. Ovarian hyperstimulation syndrome. In: Abdalla HI, Rizk B. (eds) Assisted Reproductive Technology. Abingdon, Oxford: Health Press, 1999; 37–39

76 Aboulghar MA, Mansour RT, Serour GI et al. Ultrasound guided vaginal aspiration of ascites in the treatment of ovarian hyperstimulation syndrome. Fertil Steril 1990; 53: 933–935

77 McClure N, Leya J, Radwnska E, Rawlins R, Hanning Jr RV. Luteal phase support and severe ovarian hyperstimulation syndrome. Hum Reprod 1992; 7: 597–600

78 Aboulghar MA, Mansour RT, Serour GI, Ramzy AM, Amin YM. Oocyte quality in patients with severe ovarian hyperstimulation syndrome. Fertil Steril 1997; 68: 1017–1021

79 Abramov Y, Elchalal U, Schenker JG. Obstetric outcome of in vitro fertilization pregnancies complicated by severe hyperstimulation syndrome: a multi-centre study. Fertil Steril 1998; 70: 1070–1076

*Khaldoun Sharif*

# Advances in the treatment of male factor infertility

Infertility (the inability to conceive after one year of regular unprotected intercourse) is a distressing and common condition, affecting 1 in 6 couples.[1] About 80 million couples are affected world-wide.[2] Although often viewed as the 'woman's problem', a male factor is present in 50% of couples.[3] The most severe form of male infertility is that caused by azoospermia (the total absence of sperm from the ejaculate), which is present in about 5% of all investigated infertile couples.[4] Over the past few years, major advances have occurred in the management of male factor infertility due to azoospermia. It is important for the gynaecologist to understand these advances and appreciate their clinical applications because the majority of infertile couples in most parts of the world are not managed by specialists in reproductive medicine.

## NORMAL PHYSIOLOGY

### SPERMATOGENESIS

Sperm are formed in the seminiferous tubules of the testis. Each testis is divided into an interstitial compartment (responsible for steroidogenesis) and a tubular compartment (responsible for spermatogenesis). The tubular compartment represents about 85% of the total testicular volume. Each testis is divided by connective tissue septa into about 250–300 lobules, each containing 1–3 highly convoluted seminiferous tubules. Each tubule resembles a loop draining at both ends into the rete testis, which are connected via efferent ducts into the head of the epididymis. The seminiferous tubules are surrounded by concentric layers of myofibroblasts which have the capacity of spontaneous

**Mr Khaldoun Sharif** MBBCh MRCOG MFFP MD, Consultant Obstetrician and Gynaecologist, Director of Assisted Conception Services, Birmingham Women's Hospital, Metchley Park Road, Edgbaston, Birmingham B15 2TG, UK

contraction to propel the mature sperm from the lumen of the seminiferous tubules into the rete testis.

The seminiferous tubules are lined by germinal cells (spermatogonia) and Sertoli cells. The spermatogonia are the diploid germinal cells that divide by mitosis into primary spermatocytes. These undergo a reduction division (meiosis I) into haploid secondary spermatocytes which divide (by meiosis II) into spermatids. The large spherical spermatids then undergo metamorphosis (spermiogenesis) into compact, virtually cytoplasm-free sperm with condensed DNA in the head, capped by an apical acrosome, and a tail. The developmental process from spermatogonium to sperm takes about 74 days. The human testis produces about 200–300 million sperm per day, and the entire spermatogenic process including transit time in the ductal system takes approximately three months

Sertoli cells are somatic cells located on the basement membrane of the seminiferous tubules and extend into their lumen. In a broad sense, they can be considered as the supporting structure of the germinal epithelium. Special ectoplasmic structures sustain alignment and orientation of the sperm during differentiation. Sertoli cells thus co-ordinate spermatogenesis both topographically and functionally. Each Sertoli cell is in morphological and functional contact with a defined number of sperm. This number is species-specific, and in the man is 4 sperm per Sertoli cell.

Sertoli cells have extensive cytoplasm. Where these cells come into contact with each other near the basement membrane, special occluding junctions are formed which divide the seminiferous epithelium into a basal (outer) compartment and an adluminal (inner) compartment enclosed by a functional permeability barrier, the testis–blood barrier. The mitotic division of spermatogonia takes place in the basal compartment, while the meiotic divisions of spermatocytes and spermiogenesis takes place in the adluminal compartment. Two important functions are postulated for the blood–testis barrier: (i) the physical isolation of haploid and, thereby, antigenic germ cells to prevent recognition by the immune system; and (ii) the preparation of a special milieu for the meiotic process and sperm development. Sertoli cell increase in number till the first germ cell meiotic division at puberty, which coincides with the closure of the blood–testis barrier. In adulthood, Sertoli cells are mitotically inactive.

## THE HYPOTHALAMIC–PITUITARY–TESTICULAR AXIS

Normal spermatogenesis is under the hormonal control of pituitary gonadotrophins, follicle-stimulating hormone (FSH) and luteinising hormone (LH), which are under the control of the hypothalamic gonadotrophin-releasing hormone (GnRH). LH stimulates testosterone production by the Leydig cells in the testicular interstitial compartment, and FSH stimulates the function of the Sertoli cells. Leydig cells form only 10% of the volume of the interstitial compartment, which in turn forms only 15% of the total testicular volume. However, these cells are very resistant to damage in comparison with the seminiferous tubules. For example, in cases of chemotherapy or radiotherapy-induced testicular damage, the steroidogenic ability of the testis is preserved in almost all cases despite severely reduced or absent spermatogenesis. Therefore, testosterone deficiency is usually a sign of hypogonadotrophic hypogonadism as there is inadequate stimulation of the Leydig cells. On the other hand, in testicular causes, even with very small testicular volume the testosterone level is almost always normal.

Testosterone, in addition to its endocrine actions, acts as a paracrine agent in the seminiferous tubules, where its concentration is 50 times higher than that in the peripheral circulation. Normal spermatogenesis is, therefore, dependent on the synergistic action of testosterone, LH and FSH. In the germinal epithelium, only Sertoli cells possess receptors for testosterone and FSH and the trophic effects of testosterone/FSH on gametogenesis seem to be mediated via the Sertoli cells. Testosterone and inhibin (a glycoprotein produced by Sertoli cells) exert a negative feedback action on gonadotrophin secretion. Testosterone also exerts a negative feed-back on the secretion of GnRH by the hypothalamus.

## THE SEMINAL DUCTS

The seminal ducts through which the sperm pass before reaching the prostatic urethra include the intratesticular duct system, the epididymis, the vas deferens and the ejaculatory duct. Ejaculation is characterised by the emission of the sperm and seminal plasma (which consists mainly of seminal vesicle fluid) into the prostatic urethra, the simultaneous closure of the bladder neck and the expulsion of the ejaculate. This complex process is under the control of the autonomic nervous system. Emission and bladder neck closure are under sympathetic control (thoraco-lumbar segments T9–L3). At ejaculation proper, parasympathetic fibres from the lower lumbar and upper sacral centres initiate contraction of the bulbocavernous muscles, leading to forcible ejection of ejaculate from the urethra at the same time as ascending impulses give rise to orgasm.

## CAUSES OF AZOOSPERMIA

A clinically-orientated understanding of the causes of azoospermia is recommended. In response to appropriate hormonal stimulation, the normal testis will produce sperm that are conveyed to the outside through the properly functioning and patent seminal ducts. Azoospermia can be divided into causes due to deficient hormonal stimulation of the testis (hypogonadotrophic hypogonadism), testicular dysfunction, and obstruction or dysfunction of the seminal ducts (i.e. 'pre-testicular', 'testicular', and 'post-testicular' causes). This classification, according to the level of the defect in the system, is preferred to the traditional classification of azoospermia into 'obstructive' and 'non-obstructive' causes. In that classification, the non-obstructive category contains highly treatable conditions (hypogonadotrophic hypogonadism) and untreatable cases (total testicular failure). Similarly, the obstructive category includes retrograde ejaculation, where there is actually no physical obstruction. This traditional classification can lead to lack of clarity in

**Table 11.1** Causes of azoospermia

**Pre-testicular azoospermia** (hypogonadotrophic hypogonadism)
- Congenital (Kallmann's syndrome)
- Acquired (trauma, tumours, radiotherapy, infections, drug-induced)
- Idiopathic

**Testicular azoospermia** (testicular dysfunction/failure)
- Congenital (Klinefelter's syndrome, Y chromosome deletion)
- Acquired (radiotherapy, chemotherapy, torsion, mumps orchitis)
- Developmental (testicular maldescent)
- Idiopathic (most common)

**Post-testicular azoospermia** (ductal obstruction/dysfunction)
- Ductal obstruction in:
  * Intratesticular ducts (rete testes)
  * Epididymis (post-infection, trauma, surgical damage, Young's syndrome)
  * Vas deferens (congenital bilateral absence, vasectomy, accidental damage during inguinal hernia repair)
  * Ejaculatory duct (congenital cysts, infection, trauma, urethral surgery)

- Ejaculatory dysfunction:
  * Anejaculation/retrograde ejaculation (spinal cord injury, multiple sclerosis, diabetes mellitus, bladder neck surgery, prostatectomy, sympathectomy)

patient management. The pre-testicular, testicular and post-testicular classification lends itself logically to causation, prognosis as well as clinical management. Table 11.1 presents a general outline of the classification of azoospermia.

## INITIAL ASSESSMENT OF AZOOSPERMIA

This assessment should proceed along the standard approach of history, examination and investigations. A detailed history and proper examination will contribute to the diagnosis in the majority of cases. Too often, the gynaecologist – not familiar with taking a history from men or examining them – will ignore these basic steps and miss vital clues resulting in the wrong, or even no, diagnosis and consequently offering the wrong treatment. Azoospermia is a laboratory finding and not a diagnosis.

## HISTORY

The detailed history should include the duration of infertility and whether there have been pregnancies in the past (present and previous partners), as secondary infertility will effectively exclude congenital causes. Sexual history should include frequency and adequacy of intercourse and problems with erection or libido as these are suggestive of testosterone deficiency. Diminution in beard growth and decreased frequency of shaving are other manifestations of testosterone deficiency.

**Table 11.2** History in cases of azoospermia

| History items | Relevance in azoospermia |
|---|---|
| **History of present complaint** | |
| • Type of infertility (primary, secondary) | Secondary infertility is not congenital |
| • Duration of infertility | |
| **Sexual history** | |
| • Libido | Reflects testosterone level |
| • Impotence | |
| • Frequency of intercourse | |
| **Medical history** | |
| • Recent febrile illness | Depresses spermatogenesis up to 6 months |
| • Mumps orchitis | Testicular damage |
| • Venereal disease/epididymitis | Obstruction |
| • Renal failure | Testicular failure |
| • Liver failure | Hormonal abnormality |
| • Chemotherapy/radiotherapy | Testicular damage |
| • Multiple sclerosis | Ejaculatory dysfunction |
| • Diabetes mellitus | Ejaculatory dysfunction |
| • Spinal cord injury | Ejaculatory dysfunction |
| **Surgical history** | |
| • Orchidopexy | Indicative of previous maldescent/torsion |
| • Vasectomy | Obstruction |
| • Inguinal hernia repair | Obstruction |
| • Pelvic/scrotal/urethral surgery | Ejaculatory dysfunction/obstruction |
| • Prostatectomy | Ejaculatory dysfunction |
| • Retroperitoneal surgery/sympathectomy | Ejaculatory dysfunction |
| **Testicular history** | |
| • Maldescent | Testicular damage |
| • Torsion | Testicular damage |
| • Trauma | Testicular damage |
| **Drug history** | |
| • Cimetidine | Anti-androgen |
| • Spironolactone | Anti-androgen |
| • Anabolic steroids | Inhibit pituitary gonadotrophin secretion |
| • Gonadotrophin-releasing hormone agonists | Inhibit pituitary gonadotrophin secretion |
| • Chemotherapy | Testicular damage |
| **Occupational and recreational exposure** | |
| • Pesticides/herbicides/X-ray | Testicular damage |
| • Excess heat | Testicular damage |
| • Radiation | Testicular damage |
| • Alcohol/drug abuse | Testicular damage |
| **Systems review** | |
| • Headaches/visual disturbance | Pituitary tumours |
| • Anosmia | Kallmann's syndrome |
| • Galactorrhoea | Hyperprolactinaemia |
| • Recurrent respiratory infections | Associated with Young's syndrome |
| **Previous management** | |
| • Investigations | To avoid unnecessary delay or repetition |
| • Treatment | |

Medical history should include inquiry about systemic illnesses such as multiple sclerosis, diabetes mellitus, renal failure and hepatic failure. Any recent febrile illnesses (fever exceeding 38.5°C) can depress spermatogenesis and cause testicular azoospermia up to 6 months. Past history of malignancy that required chemotherapy and radiotherapy should also be sought. Surgical history should include inquiry about orchidopexy, herniorrhaphy, retroperitoneal/pelvic surgery, and inguinal, scrotal or urethral surgery. These operations have particular relevance in cases of azoospermia (see Table 11.2). In addition, there may be a temporary depression of spermatogenesis for up to 6 months after any surgical procedure, particularly with general anaesthesia.

Particular inquiry should be made about history of testicular disorders. Minor testicular trauma is not uncommon in childhood and early adulthood (e.g. sports) and is very unlikely to cause infertility. However, it may be significant if accompanied by haematoma or haematuria and particularly if followed by testicular atrophy. Testicular torsion and testicular maldescent should be inquired about because, unless timely treated, can cause azoospermia.

Inquiry should also be made about venereal infections, orchitis and epididymitis. Mumps (parotitis) is characteristically associated with orchitis, but this occurs only in post-pubertal infections and is bilateral in only 10% of cases. Childhood mumps, post-pubertal mumps not associated with orchitis, or that leading to unilateral orchitis do not cause azoospermia. Other recognised causes of orchitis include tuberculosis, typhoid, brucellosis and syphilis. The patient would recall the history of acute orchitis as acute generalised and severe scrotal pain. Following an attack of orchitis, the recovery of fertility is variable. While some men remain azoospermic others may recover, but this can take up to 2 years. Chronic epididymitis is recalled as a recurrent localised pain or discomfort and can lead to post-testicular obstructive azoospermia. Recognised causes include chlamydia, gonorrhoea, bilharziasis, filariasis and tuberculosis.

Inquiry should also be made about exposure to drugs and environmental toxins which can affect spermatogenesis. This includes occupational exposure to X-ray, pesticides and herbicides or to medications such as sulphasalazine, cimetidine and spironolactone. Consideration needs to be given as to whether it is safe to stop the drug or whether there are any alternative preparation with no (or less) gonadotoxic effects.[5] Anabolic steroids are particularly important as they may be used by some athletes or, paradoxically, may be even prescribed by some practitioners to infertile men in the mistaken belief that they will improve sperm count. In fact, they actually act as a male contraceptive by interfering with the feedback to the pituitary gland and reducing gonadotrophin secretion.

Review of the systems should include inquiry about headaches, impaired visual fields, anosmia, galactorrhoea and recurrent respiratory infections (bronchitis, sinusitis, bronchiectasis). Any family history of male infertility or cystic fibrosis should be obtained. Finally, inquiry should be made about any previous investigations and treatment. Table 11.2 details the salient points in the history and their relevance to azoospermia.

## PHYSICAL EXAMINATION

Steps in the physical examination in cases of azoospermia are summarized in Table 11.3.

**Table 11.3** Physical examination in cases of azoospermia

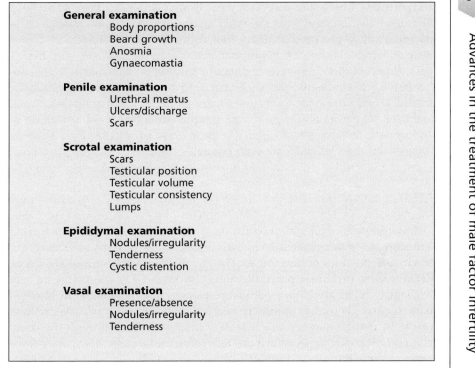

**General examination**
    Body proportions
    Beard growth
    Anosmia
    Gynaecomastia

**Penile examination**
    Urethral meatus
    Ulcers/discharge
    Scars

**Scrotal examination**
    Scars
    Testicular position
    Testicular volume
    Testicular consistency
    Lumps

**Epididymal examination**
    Nodules/irregularity
    Tenderness
    Cystic distention

**Vasal examination**
    Presence/absence
    Nodules/irregularity
    Tenderness

## GENERAL EXAMINATION

This should take place in a warm room (20–22°C) and in privacy. One of the aims of general examination is to assess if the patient is adequately androgenised. Inadequate androgenisation is indicative of testosterone deficiency, most probably resulting from pre-testicular causes. Signs of testosterone deficiency depend on the time of onset in relation to puberty.[6] If testosterone deficiency is present at the time of the normal onset of puberty, there is eunichoid tall stature because of delayed epiphyseal closure. Onset of testosterone deficiency after the normal onset of puberty does not affect body proportions, although if long-standing can lead to muscular atrophy and osteoporosis. If testosterone deficiency occurs before the normal onset of puberty there is no voice mutation, no temporal hair recession and no (or very little) beard hair growth. In addition, the upper pubic hair line remains horizontal. On the other hand, if the deficiency occurs after normal onset of puberty, the typical male hair distribution is maintained, but the sexual and body hair becomes spare, as evident by reduced frequency of beard shaving.

If general signs suggest pre-puberty onset hypogonadotrophic hypogonadism, inquire and examine for anosmia, which is a recognised sign of Kallmann's syndrome. These patients are unable to smell aromatic substances (e.g. coffee) because of a defect in the development of the olfactory lobe. However, irritant substances (e.g. ammonia) are appreciated through the trigeminal nerve and this is not affected in Kallmann's syndrome.

Gynaecomastia (increased mammary gland size in the male) is a recognised sign of Klinefelter's syndrome and the breasts should be examined by inspection and palpation. This is best done with the patient's hands placed behind his head to extend the pectoral muscles. Mild gynaecomastia is not infrequent in pubescent boys but usually disappears within 2 years. Pathological causes include various forms of hypogonadotrophic hypogonadism and hyper-prolactinaemia. Also, testicular tumours may secret human chorionic gonado-trophins (hCG) or oestrogens and lead to gynaecomastia; hence, testicular palpation and ultrasonography are essential in cases of gynaecomastia. Renal and liver failure can also cause gynaecomastia through reduced catabolism of endogenous oestrogens. Exogenous oestrogens or medications such as spironolactone and digitalis are other possible causes.

## GENITAL EXAMINATION

This is best performed with the man standing. The penis should be inspected and palpated to detect abnormally sited urethral meatus, scars, ulceration, and abnormal curvature or angulation. The site of the urethral orifice should be determined to exclude hypospadius and epispadius. These conditions are only relevant to infertility if they are severe enough (e.g. peripenile) to interfere with vaginal deposition of semen. Surgical or traumatic scars may indicate previous urethral surgery which is associated with ejaculatory dysfunction. Ulceration or discharge may indicated genital infections which may have caused obstruction.

Scrotal examination with inspection and palpation should follow. The presence of any scars should be noted. The site, size and consistency of both testes should be determined. Both should be palpable low in the scrotum. Retractile testes are those which normally lie in the scrotum but on contraction of the cremasteric muscle (in response to cold or examination) retract into the external inguinal ring. These are of no pathological significance. They can be pushed back into the scrotum during examination, which will differentiate them from true undescended testes, where incomplete descent has occurred at any point on the normal pathway of descent between the posterior abdominal wall and the scrotum. The testis, therefore, could be high scrotal (in the scrotal neck), inguinal (palpable in the inguinal canal) or intra-abdominal (impalpable). Intra-abdominal testes should be distinguished from anorchia (absent testis). Congenital anorchia is rare, occurring bilaterally in 1 in 20,000 males and unilaterally in 1 in 5000. Bilateral cases can be distinguished from abdominal testes by the hCG test, where the basal serum testosterone is measured then an hCG injection (5000 IU) is administered. In cases of anorchia there will be no rise in the testosterone level after 48–72 h, while if testes are present anywhere the levels will rise. In unilateral cases, imaging (ultrasound, computed tomography scan or magnetic resonance imaging) and if necessary surgical exploration should be used to rule out the presence of a unilateral abdominal testis. In such a case, the risk of testicular malignancy is high.

Palpation is performed to determine testicular consistency (normally rubbery) and size. Testicular volume is estimated by comparison to testis-shaped models of defined sizes (Prader orchidometer). This is done with the patient in the recumbent position because of the risk of fainting on testicular pressure. The average testicular size is 18 ml (range 12–30 ml). Small testicular size is indicative of pre-testicular or testicular causes of azoospermia. In pre-testicular causes, the testicular size is usually between 5–12 ml, with soft consistency. In Klinefelter's syndrome, the testes are typically very small (< 3 ml each) and very firm. The combination of normal testicular size and consistency with azoospermia is highly suggestive of post-testicular causes. Asymmetrical testicular consistency or size, a very hard testis or an uneven surface should raise the possibility of a testicular tumour.

The normal epididymis has a regular soft outline and is felt cranio-dorsal to the testis. Painful nodules, irregularities and induration may indicate previous infection and obstruction. Palpable cystic distention of the caput epididymis (Bayle's sign) is indicative of proximal epididymal obstruction.[7]

The vas deferens should be palpated on each side, and feels like a thin, firm cord-like structure at the neck of the scrotum. Thickened, irregular, nodular or painful vas may indicate infection and obstruction. Non-palpable vas on both sides indicate congenital bilateral absence of the vas (CBAV). Classically in CBAV, there is also normal sized testes, distended caput epididymis (due to associated absence of the lower epididymis), low volume and acidic ejaculate (due to associated agenesis of the seminal vesicles) in addition to azoospermia. However, the cord vessels may be mistaken for the vas and, in some cases, only the intra-abdominal section of the vas is absent.[8] Therefore, palpating the vas clinically does not absolutely exclude CBAV.

Examination for varicocele (distension of the pampiniform venous plexus in the spermatic cord) is by inspection and palpation. These veins will distend with increasing abdominal pressure during Valsalva's manoeuvre. Varicocele is divided into 3 grades: (i) palpable during Valsalva's manoeuvre; (ii) palpable without Valsalva's manoeuvre; and (iii) visible distension. This examination is mentioned here for completion, but, as yet, no conclusive evidence exists that varicocele causes azoospermia or male infertility, or that varicocele treatment improves fertility. Despite uncontrolled reports of benefit,[9] most controlled trials have shown no firm evidence of enhanced fertility.[10]

Examination of the prostate gland and seminal vesicles is by rectal examination. A tender or swollen prostate may indicate infection. Hardness of the prostate may be indicative of tumour, but this is rare in men presenting with infertility. The seminal vesicles are not normally palpable. Distended seminal vesicles may be indicative of ejaculatory duct obstruction (post-testicular azoospermia) and absent seminal vesicles is associated with CBAV.

Finally, the inguinal region is examined for scars which could be surgical (hernia repair) or inflammatory (tuberculosis or lymphogranuloma venereum). The presence of enlarged lymph nodes or hernias should be noted.

## INVESTIGATIONS

### CENTRIFUGATION AND SPERM PELLETING

The first step in investigating the azoospermic patient is to be certain that he has true azoospermia. The routine seminal fluid analysis is a highly subjective test,[11] and the specimen that is reported as grossly azoospermic may contain a few sperm after centrifugation (crypotozoospermia).[12] This is called sperm pelleting, where the specimen is centrifuged at 2000 rpm and the resulting pellet examined. In a study of 140 patients who were found to be azoospermic on routine semen analysis, sperm were found in 20% on sperm pelleting. This was found in men previously diagnosed as either obstructive or non-obstructive azoospermic, and irrespective of the serum FSH level or findings on previous testicular biopsy.[12] Sperm pelleting, therefore, should be performed on semen samples from all azoospermic patients. The finding of sperm will exclude total obstruction and CBAV. In addition, sperm can used for treatment.

## ANALYSIS OF POST-EJACULATION URINE

In azoospermic patients who have low volume (< 1.5 ml) ejaculate, a post-ejaculation urine specimen should be examined to rule out retrograde ejaculation.

## TRANSRECTAL ULTRASOUND (TRUS)

In the azoospermic patient with low volume ejaculate and no sperm in the post-ejaculation urine, the possibility of ejaculatory duct obstruction and seminal vesicle agenesis can be investigated with TRUS.[13] Distension of the seminal vesicles on TRUS is suggestive of ejaculatory duct obstruction, and numerous measurement criteria have been suggested. However, none of these criteria could distinguish accurately between fertile and infertile men.[14] In addition, seminal vesicle agenesis is associated with CBAV. Therefore, in current practice, TRUS is not recommended as a standard investigation for azoospermic patients with suspected seminal vesicle abnormalities.[15]

## HORMONAL MEASUREMENTS

In the azoospermic patient with no clinical hypogonadism (signs of testosterone deficiency or sexual dysfunction), measurement of serum FSH level is all that is necessary.[16] Raised levels (at least twice the upper normal limit) indicate testicular causes and are often associated with reduced testicular volume clinically. In the presence of clinical hypogonadism, the serum testosterone level should also be measured. Hypogonadotrophic hypogonadism (low FSH and testosterone) are indicative of pre-testicular causes at the pituitary or hypothalamic level. Patients with normo-gonadotrophic hypogonadism (normal FSH and low testosterone) fall into this category probably due to functional pituitary failure or pituitary tumour; only a small proportion (1%) of azoospermic men will have pre-testicular causes.[16] Rarely, the patient may have hypergonadotrophic hypogonadism (low testosterone and high FSH) indicating a testicular cause affecting both the Leydig cells and the germ cells. This can occur in some cases following childhood radiotherapy. The combination of normal FSH and normal-sized testes is highly suggestive of post-testicular causes, but about one-third of patients with this clinical picture will have testicular causes. Therefore, normal FSH does not exclude testicular causes. Serum prolactin level should be measured in cases of clinical hypogonadism, sexual dysfunction and gynaecomastia to screen for a pituitary tumour. Patients with gynaecomastia should have measurement of serum oestrogen and hCG levels also, as these hormones may be produced by adrenal or testicular tumours.

## TESTICULAR BIOPSY

The results of the investigations above allow the patients to be divided into 3 categories. The first category includes patients with hypo- or normogonado-trophic hypogonadism. These have pre-testicular causes and do not require testicular biopsy. The second category includes those with raised FSH levels, which indicate testicular causes. The aim of the management in these patients is to retrieve testicular sperm for use in intracytoplasmic sperm injection (ICSI). Testicular sperm retrieval is possible in up to 60% of these patients,[17] and is best performed where facilities are available for sperm cryopreservation. The final group are those who have normal serum FSH. Most probably the causes are post-testicular, but some will have testicular causes. Testicular biopsy is indicated in this group and should be performed where adequate microsurgical facilities are available to localise and treat possible obstruction if normal spermatogenesis is found. An intra-operative 'wet prep' cytological examination (performed by placing a small sample of fresh testicular tissue on a slide, adding a drop of Ringer's lactate, and compressing the specimen under a glass cover slip) will give immediate indication of normal spermatogenesis and indicate post-testicular causes.[18] A permanent section fixed in Bouin's solution should also be taken. If testicular causes are found (impaired spermatogenesis), then surgical sperm retrieval (with cryopreservation) should be attempted.

## SCROTAL EXPLORATION AND VASOGRAPHY

This should be done at the same time as the testicular biopsy in azoospermic patients when post-testicular causes (normal FSH, normal testicular volume, normal spermatogenesis) are suspected. The aim of this investigation is to localise the site of obstruction which could be vasal, epididymal or intra-testicular. A microscopic vasostomy and sampling of vasal fluid should be performed and, if sperm are found, then epididymal and intratesticular obstructions are excluded. A vasogram will then show if there is a vasal obstruction and its site, or if ejaculatory duct obstruction is present. Bilateral vasograms are not necessary as a unilateral patent vas is all what is necessary to rule out obstruction as the cause of azoospermia. A patent vas will indicate an ejaculatory problem.

In the absence of sperm in the vasal fluid, the epididymis is next evaluated. Dilated epididymal tubules (visible under low power magnification) are indicative of epididymal obstruction. If the epididymis is not obstructed then intratesticular obstruction should be considered.

## CHROMOSOME AND GENETIC ANALYSIS

Both structural and numerical chromosomal abnormalities are increased in azoospermic patients. Genetic testing is performed to detect these abnormalities; this will aid in the diagnosis and the genetic risk to the potential offspring to be quantified.[19]

Chromosomal analysis should be performed in azoospermic patients with testicular causes. These patients have up to 15% incidence of numerical chromosomal abnormalities, mainly Klinefelter's syndrome (47, XXY). Patients with testicular causes should also undergo screening for microdeletions in the long arm of the Y chromosome (Yq11), which have been detected in 10–15% of cases. The male children of these men will carry the same microdeletion and exhibit the same pattern of infertility in adulthood.[20] Finally, testing for cystic fibrosis transmembrane conductance regulator (CFTR) gene mutations should be performed in azoospermic men with CBAV, seminal vesicle abnormalities or low volume acidic ejaculate. These mutations are present in up to 70% of patients with CBAV and other Wolffian duct anomalies.[21]

## FURTHER MANAGEMENT

This depends on the exact cause and requires collaboration between the gynaecologist, endocrinologist and urologist. The aim is to correct the abnormality so conception can occur if possible following sexual intercourse or to retrieve surgically testicular/epididymal sperm for ICSI. With surgically retrieved sperm, ICSI has a far superior fertilisation rate to IVF (45% versus 6.9%) and consequently a higher pregnancy rate.[22]

## PRE-TESTICULAR AZOOSPERMIA

These patients represent only 1% of cases and have clinical symptoms and signs of hypogonadism, low testosterone and low (or normal) FSH. Congenital causes include Kallmann's syndrome and idiopathic hypogonadotrophic hypogonadism. Their clinical hallmark is absent or incomplete pubertal development with severe hypogonadism. Kallmann's syndrome patients will have anosmia. Acquired causes include trauma, tumours, radiotherapy, infections, and drugs (antidopaminergics). An idiopathic adult-onset hypogonadotrophic hypogonadism can also occur.[23]

All patients with hypogonadotrophic hypogonadism should be managed jointly with an endocrinologist. Serum prolactin should be measured and tests for deficiencies of other pituitary hormones (thyroid stimulation hormone, corticotrophin and growth hormone) should be performed. A neurological examination including visual field testing should be carried out and appropriate radiological examination of the pituitary fossa (computed tomography or magnetic resonance imaging) is mandatory.

In patients with normal prolactin and pituitary imaging (including Kallmann's syndrome) treatment is by testosterone replacement therapy when fertility is not desired and by pulsatile GnRH or gonadotrophins to induce fertility. One treatment protocol is to give hCG 2000 IU twice per week (Monday and Friday) for 6 months. If no normal sperm production results after that period, then human menopausal gonadotrophin is added in a dose of 150 IU three times per week (Monday, Wednesday and Friday). Normal spermatogenesis is induced in almost all patients, but it may take more than a year.[24]

In patients with raised prolactin, the commonest causes are drug induced or pituitary microadenoma. Withdrawal of the causative drug will lead to resumption of normal gonadal function. Patients with pituitary adenomas and those with raised prolactin, but normal pituitary imaging, require medical treatment with dopamine agonists (bromocriptine or cabergoline). These drugs are very effective, and neurosurgery or radiotherapy are rarely required.

## TESTICULAR AZOOSPERMIA

These patients represent about 60% of cases and present with azoospermia, usually reduced testicular volume and elevated serum FSH. Some will have normal testicular volume and FSH, and the diagnosis will be made on testicular biopsy (impaired spermatogenesis). Serum testosterone (and androgenisation) will be normal in the majority, but in some (such as Klinefelter's syndrome and testicular damage affecting the Leydig cells) there will be clinical and biochemical hypogonadism. Genetic testing, as previously discussed, will show sex chromosome numerical abnormalities in about 15% and Yq microdeletions in another 10–15%. In many, the history will indicate the primary cause of testicular dysfunction (e.g. testicular maldescent, radiotherapy, chemotherapy, torsion, mumps orchitis). Most cases, however, are idiopathic.

In recent years, major advances have been made in the management of these cases. Previously, the presence of raised serum FSH and reduced testicular volume in an azoospermic man were indications of total spermatogenic failure, so much so that the WHO manual recommended avoiding testicular biopsy in these men.[25] Sperm were thought to absent from the ejaculate because they were absent from the testis. If a single testicular biopsy did not show spermatogenesis, it was also assumed that this indicated the absence of spermatogenesis from the whole testis. Recently, two important concepts have transformed our understanding of testicular azoospermia. The first concept is the spill-over level; sperm will spill-over into the ejaculate only if they are produced at least at a minimum level in the testis. Therefore, in cases of impaired spermatogenesis, sperm may be absent from the ejaculate (i.e. azoospermia) but can still be present in the testis, albeit at a number below the spill-over level.[26] Secondly, we now recognise the focalisation of spermatogenesis. This implies that in testicular failure spermatogenesis may be present only in certain foci of seminiferous tubules, and multiple testicular sampling can lead to sperm recovery in up to 60% of cases, irrespective of testicular volume, FSH level or medical history.[26–28]

The management of these patients will include appropriate genetic testing complemented by genetic counselling.[19] Testicular sperm retrieval should then be attempted. Many techniques are available, ranging from the minimally invasive testicular fine needle aspiration (TEFNA) to multiple open testicular biopsies, which usually can be performed under local anaesthesia.[29] Sperm retrieved are used for ICSI, and lead to high fertilisation and pregnancy rates per cycle,[30] comparable to the results obtained using ejaculated sperm.[31] Regardless of the sperm origin, ultimately the pregnancy rate is dependent on the age of the female partner. In one reported series, wives of azoospermic men who were in their 20s had a 46% live birth rate per cycle, wives aged 30–36 years had a 34% live birth rate per cycle, wives aged 37–39 years had a 13% live birth rate per cycle, and wives ≥40 years had only a 4% live birth rate per cycle.[32]

## POST-TESTICULAR AZOOSPERMIA

These patients represent about 30–40% of cases and have normal testicular volume, normal serum FSH and normal spermatogenesis on testicular biopsy. Scrotal exploration and vasography (as discussed above) will localise the site of obstruction or (in the absence of obstruction) indicate an ejaculatory problem. Ductal obstruction could be found at any site; rete testis, epididymis, vas deferens or ejaculatory duct.[33]

### INTRATESTICULAR OBSTRUCTION

Obstruction in the rete testis is rare and could be caused by fibrosis or immune complex. In addition to the above findings, the vas is palpable and patent on vasography, with non-distended epididymis (the so-called 'empty epididymis syndrome'). Treatment is by testicular sperm retrieval and ICSI.

### EPIDIDYMAL OBSTRUCTION

The epididymis is by far the most common site of obstruction, particularly in the region between the upper and middle thirds. The obstruction may be congenital or acquired due to infection, trauma or surgical damage. Occasionally, it is associated with recurrent respiratory infections and sinusitis (Young's syndrome). Clinically, this type of obstruction differs from rete testis obstruction and is associated with a distended epididymis proximal to the site of obstruction (Bayle's sign). Treatment is by microsurgical vasoepididymostomy, with patency rates of 40–85% and a pregnancy rate of 30–56%.[34] Failing that, epididymal sperm could be retrieved using microsurgical epididymal sperm aspiration (MESA) or percutaneous epididymal sperm aspiration (PESA) and used for ICSI. The results are as good as those reported with ICSI using ejaculated sperm.[30,31]

### VASAL OBSTRUCTION

Non-surgical vasal obstruction (mainly due to infection) is a rare cause of obstructive azoospermia.[33] However, vasectomy is by far the commonest cause of obstruction in infertile men. For example, every year there are 100,000 patients undergoing vasectomy in the UK, and about 3% will desire fertility after the operation and seek reversal. Microsurgical vasovasostomy will give patency rates of 30–88% with a pregnancy rate of 18–53%. The longer the interval between vasectomy and reversal, the lower the pregnancy rate because of the development of seminal antisperm antibodies. In cases of failed reversal, epididymal or testicular sperm could be retrieved and used for ICSI. A few patients following technically successful reversal will have asthenozoospermia and antisperm antibodies, and spontaneous conception is less likely. ICSI with ejaculated sperm could be used in these cases.

Of patients with obstructive azoospermia, 10% will have CBAV,[33] which is frequently associated with anomalies of the lower epididymis and seminal vesicle. In 11% of men with CBAV renal agenesis is present.[35] The ejaculate will be low in volume and acidic, the vas will be impalpable clinically and the epididymal head distended. This condition is not amenable to surgical correction. Epididymal (or testicular) sperm can be retrieved and used for ICSI.[22] Of patients with CBAV, 70% are heterozygous for the CFTR gene mutation.[21] Prior to offering treatment, the cystic fibrosis (CF) carrier status should be checked. If the man is a CF carrier, then his wife should also be checked and, if she is also a carrier, there is a 25% chance of the potential offspring having CF. Pre-implantation genetic diagnosis could be offered and CF-free embryos replaced.[36]

## EJACULATORY DUCT OBSTRUCTION

Patients with ejaculatory duct obstruction will present with a picture similar to that of vasal obstruction, but the vasography will show the site of the obstruction at the ejaculatory duct. These cases may be congenital or acquired. Treatment could be transurethral resection of the duct or surgical sperm retrieval and ICSI.

## SURGICAL CORRECTION VERSUS SPERM RETRIEVAL AND ICSI IN CASES OF OBSTRUCTION

With the increasing success and simplicity of sperm retrieval methods and ICSI, there have been calls to abandon attempts at surgical correction of obstruction. However, surgical correction has many advantages over sperm retrieval and ICSI. If successful, the surgery will allow the couple to achieve further pregnancies, while a new ICSI cycle is needed for each attempt. Secondly, surgery avoids the high chance of multiple pregnancy associated with ICSI. Thirdly, performing corrective surgery may be more cost effective than sperm retrieval and ICSI.[37] Therefore, sperm retrieval/ICSI is best offered to the patient with an obstruction not amenable to surgical correction or after failed surgery.

## RETROGRADE EJACULATION

This diagnosis will be suspected in an azoospermic man because of low volume ejaculate, and confirmed by finding sperm in the post-ejaculation urine. This could be due to neurological or anatomical abnormalities. Medical causes include diabetes mellitus and surgical causes include transurethral resection of prostate, bladder neck surgery and lumbar sympathectomy. In the absence of anatomical abnormalities, a trial of medical therapy with alpha-sympathomymetics is indicated to induce antegrade ejaculation. Pseudo-ephedrine, 60 mg orally, 4 times per day is used for 2 weeks. A repeat seminal fluid analysis is then performed to see if there is antegrade ejaculation. Failure of medical treatment or retrograde ejaculation due to anatomical causes are indications for sperm retrieval for use with assisted conception methods. It is important to ensure a dilute alkaline urine for better sperm survival. The patient is given oral sodium bicarbonate 600 mg, 4 times per day beginning 2 days prior to sperm collection. The ideal pH for the specimen should be in the range of 7.5–8.5. The patient is advised to drink 300 ml of water, 1 h prior to ejaculation and then asked to first void to completion, ejaculate, and next void to completion as soon as possible after ejaculation. The post-ejaculation urine is spun down and the sperm pellet examined and processed. Depending on the count and quality of sperm collected, intra-uterine insemination, IVF or ICSI can be used.

## ANEJACULATION

Anejaculation will present with aspermia (total absence of ejaculate) and is usually caused by severe spinal cord injury or diabetes mellitus. Similar medical treatment as in retrograde ejaculation should be tried first to establish antegrade ejaculation. If that is unsuccessful, more sophisticated methods, such as vibratory stimulation or electro-ejaculation, should be tried. If these are also unsuccessful, then surgical sperm retrieval and ICSI could be used.[38]

## FUTURE ADVANCES

With the advances achieved so far, most azoospermic men now have a reason-able chance of fertility. Almost all patients with pre- and post-testicular causes can have treatment with a high prospect of success. In those with testicular causes, sperm can be retrieved in about 60%, and future advances will focus on helping the remainder. In some, round spermatids are found on testicular biopsy, and research is underway to see if these could be matured in vitro or used successfully with ICSI.[39] Another avenue for future research is to clarify further the genetic basis of male infertility and evaluate of the risk for the offspring by testing the genetic material of individual sperm.[40]

### Key points for clinical practice

- Azoospermia (the total absence of sperm from the ejaculate) is present in 5% of all infertile couples.

Normal spermatogenesis depends on adequate gonadotrophic stimulation of the testis, proper testicular function, and patent and normally functioning seminal ducts.

Azoospermia could be due to pre-testicular, testicular or post-testicular causes.

Assessment of the azoospermic patient starts by taking a detailed history and performing a full examination.

Investigations should include sperm pelleting to detect cryptozoospermia, hormonal measurements to establish the gonadotrophic status, testicular biopsy to detect spermatogenesis and vasography to look for obstruction.

Analysis of post-ejaculation urine should be performed if retrograde ejaculation is suspected because of low volume ejaculate.

Genetic testing for chromosomal abnormalities, Y chromosome microdeletion and cystic fibrosis mutations should be performed, supplemented by appropriate genetic counselling.

In patients with pre-testicular causes there is hypogonadotrophic hypogonadism. Most cases are congenital or idiopathic and are very successfully treated with hormone replacement therapy (hCG and FSH/LH). Cases due to pituitary adenomas are treated with dopamine agonists.

Patients with testicular causes are treated with surgical sperm retrieval – which is possible in 60% of them – and ICSI.

Patients with post-testicular causes due to obstruction are treated with surgical correction. In unsuccessful or unsuitable cases, surgical sperm retrieval – which is possible in almost all patients – and ICSI are used.

The treatment of patients with post-testicular causes due to ejaculatory dysfunction include medical therapy with alpha-symapthomymetics, sperm retrieval from alkaline urine, electro-ejaculation or surgical sperm retrieval and ICSI.

Close collaboration between the gynaecologist, endocrinologist and urologist is essential for the successful management of azoospermic patients.

## References

1 Hull MG, Glazener CM, Kelly NJ *et al.* Population study of causes, treatment, and outcome of infertility. BMJ 1985; 291: 1693–1697
2 World Health Organization. Achieving Reproductive Health for All. Report No. WHO/FHE/95.6. Geneva: WHO, 1995
3 World Health Organization. Towards more objectivity in diagnosis and management of male infertility. Int J Androl 1987; 7 (Suppl.): 1–53

4  Irvine DS. Epidemiology and aetiology of male infertility. Hum Reprod 1998; 13 (Suppl. 1): 33–44

5  Forman R, Gilmour-White S, Forman N. Drug-induced Infertility and Sexual Dysfunction. Cambridge: Cambridge University Press, 1996

6  Behre HM, Yeung CH, Nieschlag E. Diagnosis of male infertility and hypogonadism. In: Nieschlag E, Behre HM, (eds) Andrology. Male Reproductive Heath and Dysfunction. Berlin: Springer, 1997; 87–111

7  Bayle H. Azoospermia of excretory origin. Proc Soc Stud Fertil 1952; 4: 30–38

8  Jequier A, Ansell ID, Holmes SC. Congenital absence of the vasa deferentia presenting with infertility. J Androl 1985; 6: 15–19

9  Matthews GJ, Matthews ED, Goldstein M. Induction of spermatogenesis and achievement of pregnancy after microsurgical varicocelectomy in men with azoospermia and severe oligoasthenospermia. Fertil Steril 1998; 70: 71–75

10  Evers JLH. Varicocele. In: Templeton A, Cooke I, O'Brien PMS. (eds) Evidence-Based Fertility Treatment. London: RCOG, 1998; 109–119

11  Neuwinger J, Behre HM, Nieschlag E. External quality control in the andrology laboratory: an experimental multicentre trial. Fertil Steril 1990; 54: 308–314

12  Jaffe TM, Kim ED, Hoekstra TH, Lipshultz LI. Sperm pellet analysis: a technique to detect the presence of sperm in men considered to have azoospermia by routine semen analysis. J Urol 1998; 159: 1548–1550

13  Behre HM, Kliesch S, Schadel F, Nieschlag E. Clinical relevance of scrotal and transrectal ultrasonography in andrological patients. Int J Androl 1995; 18 (Suppl. 2): 27–31

14  Jarow JP. Transrectal ultrasonography of the infertile men. Fertil Steril 1993; 60: 1035–1039

15  Schlegel PN. Management of ejaculatory duct obstruction. In: Lipshultz LI, Howards SS. (eds) Infertility in the Male, 3rd edn. St Louis: Mosby, 1997; 385–394

16  Pandiyan N. The hormonal assessment of the infertile male. Br J Urol 1999; 83: 738–739

17  Su LM, Palermo GD, Goldstein M, Veeck LL, Rosenwaks Z, Sclegel PN. Testicular sperm extraction with intracytoplasmic sperm injection for nonobstructive azoospermia: testicular histology can predict success of sperm retrieval. J Urol 1999; 161: 112–116

18  Jow WW, Steckel J, Schlegel PN, Magid MS, Goldstein M. Motile sperm in human testis biopsy specimens. J Androl 1993; 14: 194–198

19  Mak V, Jarvi KA. The genetics of male infertility. J Urol 1996; 156: 1245–1256

20  Kim ED, Bischoff FZ, Lipshultz LI, Lamb DJ. Genetic concerns for the subfertile male in the era of ICSI. Prenat Diagn 1998; 18: 1349–1365

21  Donat R, McNeill AS, Fitzpatrick DR, Hargreave TB. The incidence of cystic fibrosis gene mutations in patients with congenital bilateral absence of the vas deferens in Scotland. Br J Urol 1997; 79: 74–77

22  Silber SJ, Nagy ZP, Liu J, Godoy H, Devroey P, Van Steirteghem AC. Conventional in-vitro fertilization versus intracytoplasmic sperm injection for patients requiring microsurgical sperm aspiration. Hum Reprod 1994; 9: 1705–1709

23  Nachtigall LB, Boepple PA, Pralong FP, Crowley WF, Jr. Adult-onset idiopathic hypogonadotropic hypogonadism – a treatable form of male infertility. N Engl J Med 1997; 336: 410–415

24  Kliesch S, Behre HM, Nieschlag E. High efficacy of gonadotropin or pulsatile gonadotropin-releasing hormone treatment in hypogonadotropic hypogonadal men. Eur J Endocrinol 1994; 131: 347–354

25  Rowe PJ, Comhaire FH, Hargreave TB, Mellows HJ. WHO manual for the standardized investigation and diagnosis of the infertile couple. Cambridge: Cambridge University Press, 1993

26  Silber SJ, Verheyen G, Goossens A, Devroey P, Van Steirteghem AC. Testicular sperm distribution in azoospermia. Fertil Steril 1998; 70(Suppl): S197

27  Silber SJ, Nagy Z, Devroey P, Tournaye H, Van Steirteghem AC. Distribution of sperm-atogenesis in the testicles of azoospermic men: the presence or absence of spermatids in the testes of men with germinal failure [published erratum in Hum Reprod 1998; 13: 780]. Hum Reprod 1997; 12: 2422–2428

28  Tournaye H, Verheyen G, Nagy P et al. Are there any predictive factors for successful testicular sperm recovery in azoospermic patients? Hum Reprod 1997; 12: 80–86

29  Westlander G, Hamberger L, Hanson C et al. Diagnostic epididymal and testicular sperm recovery and genetic aspects in azoospermic men. Hum Reprod 1999; 14: 118–122

30  Palermo GD, Schlegel PN, Hariprashad JJ *et al*. Fertilization and pregnancy outcome with intracytoplasmic sperm injection for azoospermic men. Hum Reprod 1999; 14: 741–748

31  Tarlatzis BC, Bili H. Survey on intracytoplasmic sperm injection: report from the ESHRE ICSI Task Force. European Society of Human Reproduction and Embryology. Hum Reprod 1998; 13 (Suppl. 1): 165–177

32  Silber SJ, Nagy Z, Devroey P, Camus M, Van Steirteghem AC. The effect of female age and ovarian reserve on pregnancy rate in male infertility: treatment of azoospermia with sperm retrieval and intracytoplasmic sperm injection. Hum Reprod 1997; 12: 2693–2700

33  Jaquire AM. Obstructive azoospermia: a study of 102 patients. Clin Reprod Fertil 1986; 3: 21–36

34  Schoysman R. Vaso-epididymostomy – a survey of techniques and results with considerations of delay of appearance of spermatozoa after surgery. Acta Eur Fertil 1990; 21: 239–245

35  Schlegel PN, Shin D, Goldstein M. Urogenital anomalies in men with congenital absence of the vas deferens. J Urol 1996; 155: 1644–1648

36  Ao A, Ray P, Harper J *et al*. Clinical experience with preimplantation genetic diagnosis of cystic fibrosis (delta F508). Prenat Diagn 1996; 16: 137–142

37  Wolter S, Neubauer S, Heidenreich A. Vasovasostomy versus MESA/TESE combined with ICSI – a cost benefit analysis. J Urol 1999; 161 (Suppl. 4): 312

38  Dahlberg A, Ruutu M, Hovatta O. Pregnancy results from a vibrator application, electroejaculation, and a vas aspiration programme in spinal-cord injured men. Hum Reprod 1995; 10: 2305–2307

39  Prapas Y, Chatziparasidou A, Vanderwalmen P *et al*. Spermatid injection. Hum Reprod 1999; 14: 2186–2188

40  Moosani N, Pattinson HA, Carter MD, Cox DM, Rademaker AW, Martin RH. Chromosomal analysis of sperm from men with idiopathic infertility using sperm karyotyping and fluorescence *in situ* hybridization. Fertil Steril 1995; 64: 811–817

*Edward P. Morris  Janice Rymer*

# Update on the risk–benefit ratio of hormone replacement therapy in the menopause

The population is ageing and, therefore, the number of postmenopausal women is increasing. The medical profession now diverts an increasing amount of attention to alleviating both the symptoms experienced by women during the menopause and the long-term effects of oestrogen deficiency in women. Symptomatology can be divided into three categories: (i) vasomotor; (ii) psychological; and (iii) urogenital/sexual. Longer term effects of the menopause include increased bone loss which may lead to osteoporosis and an increase in the risk of cardiovascular disease.

The menopause is an 'oestrogen deficient state' and it is thus logical to conclude that oestrogen replacement therapy should correct the problems. Due to the increased risk of endometrial cancer, non-hysterectomised women should not be administered oestrogen in isolation. The use of progestogens is widely accepted to counteract unwanted endometrial stimulation, but effects on risk markers for cardiovascular disease suggests that progestogens may blunt some of the beneficial effects of oestrogen.[1]

The last decade has seen many advances in the management of the menopause – both in the drugs administered and the routes of administration. Few areas of medicine have such a diversity of therapeutic options. The place of both new and old therapies will be evaluated in this review – using mainly randomised controlled trials and systematic reviews. Non-randomised and other controlled trials will only be included where there are no adequate randomised controlled trials.

**Dr Edward P. Morris** BSc MBBS MRCOG, Specialist Registrar and Honorary Lecturer, Guy's, King's and St Thomas' Medical School, HRT Research Unit, Guy's Hospital, London SE1 9RT, UK (for correspondence)

**Dr Janice Rymer** MBChB MD MRCOG FRNZCOG, Senior Lecturer and Consultant, Department of Obstetrics and Gynaecology, Guy's, King's and St Thomas' Medical School, 7th Floor North Wing, St Thomas' Hospital, London SE1 7EH, UK

Menopause is diagnosed once 12 months have elapsed since the final menstrual period. This definition is not particularly useful as it is retrospective. The perimenopause is clinically more relevant because it encompasses the phase commencing with the onset of oestrogen deficiency symptoms and extends to 1 year after the last menstrual period. The perimenopause, or 'menopausal transition', covers the phase from ovulatory cycles with well-characterised hormone profiles to ovarian failure demonstrated by low oestrogen and high gonadotrophin levels. The average age of women at the menopause is 50 years and 9 months, but the perimenopause has a median age at onset of 45.5–47.5 years and an average duration of 4 years. The primary endocrine event in reproductive ageing may be a fall in inhibin B, allowing follicle stimulating hormone (FSH) to rise which, in turn, leads to accelerated follicle development and increased oestrogen secretion until the follicle pool has been exhausted.[2] Autopsy, oophorectomy studies, and mathematical models[3] have all indicated that the rate of follicular depletion increases during the menopausal transition, and accelerated follicular development of recruited follicles is also observed.

## VASOMOTOR SYMPTOMS

The commonest symptoms of the perimenopause are: hot flushes, night sweats, palpitations, and headaches that are due to vasomotor instability and affect 80% of women. The aetiology of the vasomotor symptoms is complex and remains uncertain, but is possibly due to lability of the thermoregulatory centre in the hypothalamus induced by falling oestrogen and progesterone levels.

## PSYCHOLOGICAL SYMPTOMS

The link between psychological symptoms and the perimenopause remains uncertain and whether the development of these symptoms depends upon psychosocial influences. A recognised increase in depressive symptoms occurs during the perimenopause, but there is little evidence to support an increase in the incidence of clinical depression. It is, therefore, important to distinguish between depressed mood and clinical depression using recognised diagnostic techniques. The highest frequency of depression occurs in the 30–45 year age range and, at present, no firm data support the view that natural menopause causes depression.[4]

Recognised symptoms include mood swings, anxiety, depressed mood, decreased libido, insomnia, irritability, forgetfulness, poor concentration and fatigue. Such symptoms are common in all women, both pre- and postmenopausal, and are also frequently associated with other psychiatric illnesses. Many of the published studies have used selected populations, e.g. hospital clinic attendees, and these women may be different in their behaviour, personality, and symptom profile from women of the same age who do not seek medical advice. Population-based studies have shown that about 20% perimenopausal women have depressed mood as a central problem. The interplay between biological changes associated with ovarian failure and the psychosocial changes occurring at this time is complex. Some groups attribute mood changes to the former[5] and some to the latter.[6]

## UROGENITAL SYMPTOMS AND LIBIDO

The predominant lower genital tract symptoms precipitated by the oestrogen deficiency of the menopause are urinary incontinence and vaginal dryness. Stress incontinence is the commonest form of incontinence; however, most women have a combination of bladder problems. This is likely to be due to the presence of oestrogen receptors in the tissues of the bladder, urethra, and muscles of the pelvic floor. Hence, oestrogen deficiency may be an aetiological factor in the development of urinary incontinence. Symptoms of vaginal dryness such as irritation, discharge, bleeding and dyspareunia lead to significant morbidity. The effect of such symptoms on the patient can be assessed using symptom scores and can be demonstrated objectively by measuring cellularity via the karyopyknotic index from vaginal smears, which reflects the oestrogen status of the vagina.

Addressing the subject of sexuality in the postmenopausal woman is more complex as the proportional influence of the various female hormones on sexual drive is incompletely understood, as is the influence of psychological, vasomotor and other menopausal symptoms. Loss of oestrogen can affect sexual drive through its effects on vaginal moisture alone, as women may find intercourse uncomfortable, if not painful. Loss of testosterone also accompanies natural menopause, but at a rate slower than oestrogen decline. Testosterone loss is significantly quicker in women with a surgically induced menopause and women may become symptomatic sooner, often requiring testosterone replacement in combination with oestrogen replacement therapy.

## CARDIOVASCULAR DISEASE

It has long been accepted that the menopausal years are associated with a sharp increase in deaths from cardiovascular disease (CVD) in women – with mortality increasing to a higher rate than experienced by the premenopausal population – to a point where the deaths in women equal and then exceed those of men. Until recently the accepted explanation of this was that women lose the cardioprotective effect of oestrogen at the menopause. It has been suggested recently that no sudden increase in CVD death rates follow the menopause and that the female death rate continues to rise, as in men, and contrary to popular belief it neither catches up, nor overtakes the male CVD death rates.[7] The main conclusion from this author was that the increase of CVD death rates at the menopause is 'a myth' that has been based on incorrect interpretation of mortality. This may explain why the benefits of hormone replacement therapy (HRT) on the cardiovascular system may not be as great as suggested by the early epidemiological studies.

It would seem hard to ignore the apparently pro-atherogenic serum lipid and lipoprotein changes and changes in other surrogate markers for CVD that accompany the menopause. For this reason, many aspects of CVD in the menopause require further research.

## OSTEOPOROSIS

Women reach their peak bone mass in their twenties, followed by a plateau until their forties when there is age related bone loss (as with men); then, with ovarian failure, there is an accelerated phase of bone loss. At the time of declining ovarian function, there is a rapid increase in bone formation and resorption, with bone resorption exceeding formation. This apparent uncoupling of the normal balance of bone turnover results in a net loss of bone calcium.

Osteoporosis is associated with high morbidity and mortality. The mortality is estimated at more than 20% at 1 year following a fractured hip. In addition, women may lose their independence, thus significantly reducing their quality of life. The estimated annual financial cost to the NHS in the UK of osteoporosis related illness is estimated to be in the order of £900 million.

## BENEFITS

### OESTROGEN

The common forms of available oestrogen are conjugated equine oestrogen (Premarin; Wyeth), and oestradiol, either as 17β-oestradiol or oestradiol valerate. Conjugated oestrogen is available as an oral preparation or topical cream only. Oestradiol is available as many different formulations – oral, transdermal patches, gels, implant pellets and topical creams. Most large-scale and long-term studies with oestrogen have used oral conjugated oestrogen. There is little long–term data of the effects of oestradiol from large randomised studies.

#### Vasomotor symptoms
The efficacy of oestrogen in alleviating menopausal symptoms is well established. Most clinical data originate from either large-scale epidemiological studies or randomised controlled studies involving evaluations of one preparation against the next. There is a clear benefit of oestrogen therapy on vasomotor symptoms; most studies having a duration of 12 months on average. More recently, a 3 year randomised trial of oestrogen and various oestrogen/progestogen regimens versus placebo[8] confirmed a clear reduction in vasomotor symptoms of 72% to 83% at 12 months when compared to placebo, an effect that was significantly reduced by 3 years. This apparent loss of treatment effect was probably due to the reduction in the numbers of women experiencing vasomotor symptoms as the menopause progresses rather than a tolerance to the effects of oestrogen.

#### Psychological symptoms
A recent meta-analysis concluded that oestrogen was effective in reducing depressed mood amongst menopausal women.[9] There is no evidence from

randomised trials confirming that oestrogen either elevates mood or is effective in treating clinically proven depression. Observational studies suggest that there may be a beneficial effect of oestrogen on cognitive function, both in women with and without Alzheimer's disease. Randomised trials are awaited in these interesting areas.

## Urogenital symptoms and libido

Oestrogen replacement contributes to the return of improved cell turnover and lubrication of the postmenopausal genital tract – a phenomenon known as oestrogenisation. This stimulation is considered harmful in the uterus when oestrogen is administered unopposed by progesterone. With regard to the lower genital tract, most evidence for improved oestrogenisation with administration of oestrogen comes from observational and case control studies. However, a recent meta-analysis[10] demonstrated that oestrogen is effective in improving the oestrogenisation of the lower genital tract, regardless of the route of administration.

Whether oestrogenisation of the lower genital tract improves incontinence is uncertain. Most research in this area addresses treatment of incontinence rather than prevention. Two recent meta-analyses[11,12] have shown that there is a significant effect of oestrogen replacement on subjective measures of symptomatology with no effect on objective measures of incontinence. These authors concluded that larger randomised trials are needed.

The issue of whether oestrogen replacement alone improves libido and sexual life is incompletely understood. The effect of improving oestrogenisation of the genital tract aids lubrication and elasticity of the vagina, thus reducing experience of significant dyspareunia. This in itself can improve postmenopausal sexual relationships. As effective oestrogenisation can easily be achieved using topical routes with minimal unwanted effects, this is an excellent first-line therapy. There is no evidence to support a direct effect of oestrogen on libido.

## Cardiovascular disease

Administration of oestrogen to the postmenopausal woman has been shown to be effective in the primary prevention of CVD risk in most observational studies, as shown by a recent meta-analysis.[13] The potential reduction in CVD risk is up to 30%, though results from larger, long-term randomised trials are awaited.

Secondary prevention of CVD, if data from primary prevention studies could be extrapolated to those with pre-existing CVD, could also be considered an indication for oestrogen replacement. With the recent publication of the HERS study,[14] which concluded that oestrogen replacement did not reduce the number of deaths in those with pre-existing CVD, there is doubt in this area. This study has attracted both support and criticism. Support comes from those who feel that such a large study has been carefully performed, showing no effect of secondary prevention of CVD whilst demonstrating the beneficial lipid changes that many feel reduces CVD risk. Criticism appears to be mainly focused around the use of medroxyprogesterone acetate as the progesterone used and the premature end to the study, which has significantly impaired the study's potential to observe a beneficial effect of oestrogen over time.

## Osteoporosis

Oestrogen replacement is widely accepted to have a significant, beneficial effect

Update on the risk–benefit ratio of hormone replacement therapy in the menopause on the postmenopausal female skeleton. Supportive data are available from observational, case-control and randomised studies comparing various oestrogen preparations against placebo or against each other using biochemical markers and quantitative measures of bone density.[15] Oestrogen appears to reduce the presentation of fractures at clinically relevant sites, such as the spine and neck of femur, by 50% and 30%, respectively.[16,17]

## PROGESTOGENS

There are many different available progestogens – the commonest available being norethisterone, medroxyprogesterone acetate and levonorgestrel. The study of the effect of these compounds alone in the context of the menopause is difficult, as most investigations involve the administration of oestrogen alongside progestogens.

### Vasomotor symptoms

Progestogens have been demonstrated to be effective therapies for the treatment of menopausal symptoms. Unfortunately, to achieve a good clinical effect, relatively high doses are needed; with the lowest dose used being 20 mg medroxyprogesterone acetate (MPA) per day. Most studies have a duration of less than 12 months and show significant reductions in experienced vasomotor symptoms.[18–22]

### Psychological symptoms, urogenital tract, libido and cardiovascular disease

The principal desired effect of progesterone on the genital tract is its ability to prevent oestrogenic stimulation of the endometrium, similar to its physiological role in the menstrual cycle. When giving HRT to postmenopausal women, at least 12 days of progestogen is required to induce cyclical bleeding in perimenopausal or menopausal women. Continuous low dose progestogen is adequate for prevention of endometrial stimulation thus avoiding monthly bleeds – so-called 'period free' HRT.

No evidence suggests any benefit of progestogens on psychological symptoms, the lower genital tract and libido. Some evidence suggests possible harm, as discussed below.

### Osteoporosis

Progestogens alone in the absence of oestrogen have been shown to inhibit bone loss.[23–25] Norethisterone in doses of 10 mg daily has been shown to reduce bone loss in postmenopausal women,[26], although smaller doses of norethisterone (up to 3.5 mg) did not appear to prevent bone loss. The effect of these alterations on the incidence of fracture has not been investigated. Norethisterone is an androgenic progestogen and there is little evidence to suggest that other progestogens, such as medroxyprogesterone acetate or micronised progesterone, increase bone density.

## TIBOLONE

Tibolone (Livial; Organon) has oestrogenic, progestogenic and androgenic properties, both as a parent compound, and via its metabolites which have varying affinities for the oestrogen, progesterone and androgen receptors.[27] Evidence suggests that the site of metabolism of the drug contributes to its 'tissue specific' action, for example at the endometrium there is a predominance of the Δ-4 isomer.[28] This effect is what contributes to the drug's period-free action.

### Vasomotor symptoms

Tibolone demonstrates a significantly beneficial effect on vasomotor symptoms, equivalent to oestrogen[29] and significantly better that placebo.[30]

### Psychological symptoms

No evidence supports an effect of tibolone on depression, but an early study showed a beneficial effect on mood and insomnia.[30]

### Urogenital tract and libido

This drug has been shown in observational and case-control studies to improve both libido and oestrogenisation of the lower genital tract.[27,31] One randomised trial has shown a beneficial effect of tibolone on subjective reports of sexual enjoyment and vaginal lubrication.[32] In another randomised trial in which tibolone was compared to continuous combined oestrogen and progesterone, there was a significant improvement in sexual enjoyment and frequency in those on tibolone in comparison to a group taking combined oestrogen.[33] We found no trials demonstrating effects on urinary incontinence.

### Cardiovascular disease

Tibolone appears to have a largely oestrogenic effect on markers of CVD with reductions in total triglycerides, total cholesterol,[34] and lipoprotein a.[35] Low density lipoprotein (LDL) cholesterol is unaltered and high density lipoprotein (HDL) cholesterol is reduced. Though a reduction in HDL cholesterol is potentially undesirable, the implications of these changes on CVD risk are unclear, especially in the light of recent evidence from vessel wall studies in animals[36] and humans[37] that suggest either a neutral or even a protective effect of tibolone on the cardiovascular system.

### Osteoporosis

Tibolone prevents bone loss in recently postmenopausal women[38] and in women with established osteoporosis.[39]

## RALOXIFENE

Raloxifene (Evista; Eli Lilly) belongs to the benzothiaphene family of drugs and is also part of an expanding class of drugs known as selective oestrogen receptor modulators (SERMS). This selective action on the oestrogen receptor involves both drug and tissue specific agonism or antagonism of the oestrogen receptor. In all susceptible tissues, pure oestrogens stimulate whereas pure anti-oestrogens, such as ICI 182 780 (Zeneca), antagonise the oestrogen receptor. Raloxifene, therefore, demonstrates selective action or tissue specificity with oestrogenic or anti-oestrogenic activity – depending on the target tissue. A complete explanation for these varying effects has yet to be discovered. An interplay of factors may occur such as local oestrogen metabolites, novel oestrogen receptors, multiple transcriptional activating functions such as AF-1 and AF-2[40], differing ligand-induced receptor conformations,[41] or possibly modulation of cellular function via a novel pathway induced by the raloxifene-receptor conformation; the so-called 'raloxifene response element'.[42]

In the UK, raloxifene is currently licensed solely for the prevention of non-traumatic vertebral fractures in postmenopausal women at increased risk of osteoporosis.

### Vasomotor symptoms, psychological symptoms, urogenital tract and libido
No information suggests that raloxifene has any beneficial effects on vasomotor symptoms, psychological symptoms, the lower genital tract and libido. Potential adverse effects in these areas are discussed below.

The earliest study into the long term effects of raloxifene[43] ($n$ = 601) compared the marketed dose of 60 mg of raloxifene per day against placebo and reported no significant differences between the 60 mg dose of raloxifene per day and placebo groups in either transvaginal ultrasound assessed endometrial thickness or vaginal bleeding rates (3.0% raloxifene versus 2.2% placebo). Other studies since have confirmed that raloxifene does not stimulate the endometrium, therefore confirming that it has a period-free action.

### Cardiovascular disease
A potentially beneficial effect of raloxifene on the cardiovascular system has been demonstrated in clinical trials analysing the effects on serum lipids.[43] A more detailed study into the effects of raloxifene on serum lipids[44] was performed in 390 women randomised to receive either placebo, raloxifene 60 mg daily, raloxifene 120 mg daily or conventional HRT (continuous combined equine oestrogen 0.625 mg and medroxyprogesterone acetate 2.5 mg daily). The following comparisons with the effects of HRT were made: after 6 months, raloxifene was found to reduce serum levels of LDL-C to the same extent as HRT; lipoprotein a was reduced by 7%, whereas HRT produced a 19% reduction; there were also significant increases in HDL-C in both groups with HRT again producing the greater effect; serum triglycerides increased significantly in the HRT group with no demonstrable increase in the raloxifene treated women.

### Osteoporosis
In the 601 women in the study discussed above, there was a significant reduction in biochemically assessed bone turn-over. This resulted in a modest, but statistically significant, increase in bone density over 2 years in the lumbar spine as assessed by bone densitometry (mean 1.6% increase from baseline, raloxifene versus 0.8% decrease, placebo). The MORE study (Multiple Outcomes of Raloxifene Evaluation) is a double-blind, placebo-controlled trial of 7705 osteoporotic women randomised to either placebo or raloxifene at a dose of 60 mg or 120 mg per day which has recently undergone a 2 year interim analysis. This showed the risk of vertebral fracture over 2 years fell by 44% in raloxifene users when compared to placebo ($P < 0.001$).[45]

# PHYTO-OESTROGENS

Phyto-oestrogens are compounds derived from plants that demonstrate mild oestrogenic activity – only about 2% that of oestradiol. The commonest types are coumestans, lignans, and isoflavones. The most oestrogenically potent are the isoflavones, two of which are genisten and daidzien. These are found almost exclusively in soya, chick peas, lentils, and peas. Most preparations in this area are marketed as food supplements in bread, snack bars or health drinks. The efficacy of these drugs is hard to study as standards of potency and bioavailability vary considerably from one preparation to another. As a consequence, there are no randomised controlled trials.

## Symptoms

At present, no randomised controlled studies exist to confirm that this group of compounds is effective in the treatment of the group of symptoms that accompanies the menopause. In the few studies that are available, phyto-oestrogens may have a role in alleviating menopausal symptoms related to oestrogen deficiency.[46] This effect may be of significant benefit to women who do not wish to take pharmacological preparations, instead preferring the more natural approach that accompanies these plant extracts.

## Osteoporosis and cardiovascular disease

No evidence is available to suggest that this group of drugs is effective in the prevention or treatment of osteoporosis, or the prevention or cardiovascular disease.

## RISKS

## OESTROGEN

In the initial years of HRT prescribing, it became clear that the long-term administration of oestrogen to non-hysterectomised women is associated with endometrial stimulation which, in severe cases, resulted in endometrial carcinoma. Though the issue of oestrogenic endometrial stimulation remains, it is now clear that concomitant administration of progestogen, either cyclically or continuously, can virtually eliminate the risk of developing oestrogen-induced endometrial adenocarcinoma.

Breast cancer is without doubt the most feared cancer by women. In the UK, women have a 1 in 12 life-time risk of developing the disease and a 1 in 26 risk of dying from it.[47] For many years, there have been studies suggesting an adverse effect of oestrogen on breast cancer risk and, until recently, there has been confusion as to the exact degree of increased risk accompanying HRT use. This issue was recently clarified in a large multicentre re-analysis of existing data of breast cancer sufferers and HRT use.[48] The investigators showed that oestrogen use was associated with a 2.3% per year increase in risk of developing breast cancer which was approximately equivalent to the 2.8% increase per year associated with a naturally delayed menopause. They presented that, in women aged 50–70 years, the natural risk of developing breast cancer was 45:1000 which increases to 47:1000 with 5 years of HRT use, 51:1000 with 10 years and 57:1000 after 15 years of HRT. They also confirmed the findings of other investigators that, if a woman were to develop breast cancer whilst on HRT, she had a significantly lower chance of dying from the disease.

Thrombo-embolic disease (TED) has long been associated with the oestrogens in the oral contraceptive pill, and the effect of the biologically less potent oestrogens contained in HRT on TED risk has long been questioned. Recently, several studies[49–51] have demonstrated an increase in risk of developing TED in the region of 2–4-fold. This was confirmed in the HERS study, a large randomised placebo-controlled study of women taking conjugated oestrogens.[14] Though this effect is statistically significant, it is important to be aware that, in clinical practice, this means that risk of developing TED increases from 1:10,000 to 3:10,000 women. In the consulting room, this means little for the fit, healthy woman without a history of TED. For those with a clear history of TED, it is important to inform them of the increased risks associated with oestrogens, and to establish any significant family history suggesting an inherited thrombophilia, which should then be screened for prior to commencing HRT.

## PROGESTOGENS

It is difficult to separate the contribution of unwanted effects caused by progestogens from the potential unwanted effects of oestrogen as these drugs are usually administered alongside oestrogen to prevent endometrial stimulation. Progestogens are commonly blamed for producing depression, weight gain, bloating and adversely affecting serum lipids.

Two recent randomised controlled trials have shown that the unwanted effects of progestogens alongside oestrogen in common preparations may not be as severe as initially thought. In 321 hysterectomised women taking conjugated oestrogens, one group randomised to take continuous norgestrel and one to placebo daily, there was no difference in symptoms between the groups, especially in weight gain and bloating.[52] This study also showed that progesterone appeared to blunt some of the beneficial effects of oestrogen on the lipid profile. The well publicised Postmenopausal Estrogen/Progestin Interventions (PEPI) study compared various oestrogen-progestogen regimens and their effect on many outcomes over 3 years in 875 women.[8] The only symptom that increased significantly with the addition of progestogen was an increase in breast discomfort. There was a measurable effect of progestogens on serum lipids – again blunting the effects of oestrogen. The overall conclusion from the PEPI study was that it is still better to give progestogens with oestrogens than nothing at all.

It is important to be aware that both the above highly relevant studies have analysed progestogens with conjugated equine oestrogens. Large randomised studies with oestradiol are lacking.

## TIBOLONE

The unwanted effects of this drug include greasiness of the skin and an increase in hair growth, both of which are androgenic effects.[27] As with most 'period free' HRT preparations, this drug also has a small incidence of 10–20% of breakthrough bleeding in the long-term. Small amounts of bleeding in the first 6 months of therapy are considered normal in the absence of other clinical signs and usually stop with time. There is no evidence to suggest an increase in the incidence of TED with tibolone. No large, randomised, clinical data are available to asses effects on the breast, but there is early in vitro and small clinical study data that suggest that it may have a beneficial effect on breast tissue.[27]

## RALOXIFENE

Raloxifene does not treat hot flushes and evidence shows that it may worsen them.[43,44] As with oestrogen, evidence from pooled data shows that raloxifene increases the risk of VTE. The relative risk compared to placebo is approximately 2.5. Leg cramps are experienced by approximately 5.5% of women taking raloxifene. As vaginal bleeding is an unexpected outcome on raloxifene, any such episodes should be investigated.

## PHYTO-OESTROGENS

It is difficult to identify clearly the risks of phyto-oestrogens due to the enormous diversity of preparations. It comes as significant concern to many gynaecologists that drugs with oestrogenic activity are being administered to postmenopausal women with a uterus – thus potentially exposing them to an unquantifiable increased risk of endometrial carcinoma. It must also be assumed that, until the manufacturers of these drugs standardise potencies of these preparations and perform randomised controlled trials, these compounds must also attract other unwanted effects such as stimulation of the breast.

## CONCLUSION

HRT does not suit everyone. Each woman needs to be aware of the benefits and potential risks of HRT so that she can make an informed decision. Our duty as clinicians is to ensure that women are provided with consistent and up-to-date information.

## THE FUTURE

The new millennium will be an exciting time for those working with meno-pausal patients. Oestrogen will continue to be used for the prevention of unwanted sequelae of the menopause. Large randomised controlled trials are in progress to provide answers regarding HRT and the prevention of cardio-vascular disease, Alzheimer's disease, and long-term morbidity and mortality.

Will the new millennium provide the long awaited 'ideal' replacement therapy – a drug that prevents vasomotor symptoms, prevents osteoporosis, does not stimulate the endometrium or breast, protects the woman from cardiovascular disease and makes her feel well with improved quality of life?

# Key points for clinical practice

- Proper management of the health issues surrounding the menopause is important to reduce morbidity from the symptoms of the menopause and mortality in the longer term from bone loss and cardiovascular disease.

- Evidence to support the use of HRT for the treatment of menopausal symptoms and prevention of osteoporosis is convincing.

- We await data from larger studies concerning improvements in cardiovascular risk with HRT.

- Novel drugs, such as SERMs, should considered only for patients who are at risk of osteoporotic fracture and do not wish to take HRT.

- The effects of drug groups, such as clonidine, phyto-oestrogens and progestogens, may be suitable for some women, but prescribers should be aware that there is considerably less data with these compounds than with oestrogen alone.

- Venous thrombo-embolic disease is increased 3-fold with oestrogen administration and caution should be taken when prescribing oestrogen to women at risk.

- The excess risk of breast cancer with HRT is small, especially when it is considered that few women take HRT for extended periods of time.

- The increase in breast cancer is, however, an inevitable part of the consultation when prescribing HRT and practitioners should have the correct statistics to reassure the patient.

- Adherence with therapy is traditionally poor in the UK. Increasing use of HRT depends on many factors, including the correct choice of drug, minimising unwanted effects and a trusting, healthy dialogue between doctor and patient.

## References

1 The Writing Group for the PEPI Trial. Effects of estrogen or estrogen/progestin regimens on heart disease risk factors in postmenopausal women. JAMA 1995; 273: 199–208

2 Pellicer A, Simon C, Mari M *et al*. Effects of aging on the on the human ovary: the secretion of immunoreactive aaa-inhibin and progesterone. Fertil Steril 1994; 61: 663–668

3 Teede H, Burger HG. The menopausal transition. In: Studd J. (ed) The Management of the Menopause. London: Parthenon, 1998; 1–12

4 Nicol-Smith L. Causality, menopause and depression: a critical review of the literature. BMJ 1996; 313: 1129–1132

5 Holte A. Influence of natural menopause on health complaints: a prospective study of healthy Norwegian women. Maturitas 1992; 14: 127–141

6 Kaufert P, Gilbert P, Tate R. The Manitoba project: a re-examination of the link between menopause and depression. Maturitas 1992; 14: 143–155

7 Tunstal-Pedoe H. Myth and paradox of coronary risk and the menopause. Lancet 1998; 351: 1425–1427

8 Greendale GA, Reboussin BA, Hogan P *et al*. Symptom relief and side effects of postmenopausal hormones: results from the postmenopausal estrogen/progestin

interventions trial. Obstet Gynecol 1998; 92: 982–988

9  Zweifel JE, O'Brien WH. A meta-analysis of the effect of HRT upon depressed mood. Psychoneuroendocrinology 1997; 22: 189–212

10  Cardozo L, Bachmann G, McClish D, Fonda DLB. Meta-analysis of estrogen therapy in the management of urogenital atrophy in postmenopausal women: second report of the Hormones and Urogenital Therapy Committee. Obstet Gynecol 1998; 92: 722–727

11  Fantl JA, Cardozo L, McClish DK. Estrogen therapy in the management of urinary incontinence in postmenopausal women: first report of the Hormones and Urogenital Therapy Committee. Obstet Gynecol 1994; 83: 12–18

12  Zullo MA, Oliva C, Falconi G, Paparella P, Mancuso S. Efficacy of the estrogen therapy against urinary incontinence. A meta-analysis. Minerva Ginecol 1998; 50: 199–205

13  Barrett-Connor E, Grady D. Hormone replacement therapy, heart disease and other considerations. Annu Rev Public Health 1998; 18: 55–72.

14  Hulley S, Grady D, Bush T *et al*. Randomized trial of estrogen plus progestin for secondary prevention of coronary heart disease in postmenopausal women. JAMA 1998; 280: 605–613

15  Fogelman I. The effects of oestrogen deficiency on the skeleton and its prevention. Br J Obstet Gynaecol 1996; 103: 5–9

16  Grady D, Rubin SM, Petitti DB *et al*. Hormone therapy to prevent disease and prolong life in postmenopausal women. Ann Intern Med 1992; 117: 1016–1037

17  Lufkin EG, Wahner HW, O'Fallon WM *et al*. Treatment of postmenopausal osteoporosis with transdermal estrogen. Ann Intern Med 1992; 119: 1–9

18  Loprinzi CL, Michalak JC, Quella SK *et al*. Megestrol acetate for the prevention of hot flushes. N Engl J Med 1994; 331: 347–352

19  Lobo RA, McCormick W, Singer F, Roy S. DMPA compared with conjugated oestrogens for the treatment of postmenopausal women. Obstet Gynecol 1984; 63: 1–5

20  Aslaksen K, Frankendal B. Effect of oral MPA on menopausal symptoms on patients with endometrial carcinoma. Acta Obstet Gynecol Scand 1982; 61: 423–428

21  Schiff I, Tulchinsky D, Cramer D, Ryan KJ. Oral MPA in the treatment of postmenopausal symptoms. JAMA 1980; 244: 1443–1445

22  Bullock JL, Massey FM, Gambrell RD. Use of MPA to prevent menopausal symptoms. Obstet Gynecol 1975; 46: 165–168

23  Erlik Y, Medrum DR, Lagasse LD, Judd HL. Effect of megestrol acetate on flushing and bone metabolism in post-menopausal women. Maturitas 1981; A3: 167–172

24  Mandel FP, Davidson BJ, Erlik Y, Judd HL, Meldrum DR. Effects of progestins on bone metabolism in post-menopausal women. J Reprod Med 1982; 13: 511–514

25  Abdalla HI, Hart DM, Lindsay R, Leggate I, Hooke A. Prevention of bone mineral loss in postmenopausal women by norethisterone. Obstet Gynecol 1985; 66: 789–792

26  Horowitz M, Wishart J, Need AG, Morris H, Philcox J, Nordin BE. Treatment of postmenopausal hyperparathyroidism with norethindrone. Arch Intern Med 1987; 147: 681

27  Rymer JM. The effects of tibolone. Gynaecol Endocrinol 1998; 12: 213–220

28  Markiewicz L, Gurpide E. In vitro evaluation of estrogenic, estrogenic antagonistic and progestagenic effects of a steroidal drug (Org OD14) and its metabolites on human endometrium. J Steroid Biochem 1990; 35: 535–541

29  Milner MH, Sinnott MM, Cooke TM *et al*. A two year study of lipid and lipoprotein changes in postmenopausal women with tibolone and estrogen-progestin. Obstet Gynecol 1996; 87: 593–599

30  Kicovic PM, Cortes-Prieto J, Luisi M, Milojevic S, Franchi F. Placebo-controlled cross-over study of effects of Org OD14 in menopausal women. Reproduccion 1982; 6: 81–91

31  Rymer J, Chapman M, Fogelman I, Wilson POG. A study into the effect of tibolone on the vagina in postmenopausal women. Maturitas 1994; 18: 127–133

32  Hammar M, Christau S, Nathorst-Boos J, Rud T, Garre K. A double-blind, randomised trial comparing the effects of tibolone and continuous combined hormone replacement therapy in postmenopausal women with menopausal symptoms. Br J Obstet Gynaecol 1998; 105: 904–911

33  Nathorst-Boos J, Hammar M. Effect on sexual life – a comparison between tibolone and a continuous estradiol-norethisterone acetate regimen. Maturitas 1997; 26: 15–20

34 Bjarnason NH, Bjarnason K, Haarbo J, Coelingh Bennink HJT, Christiansen C. Tibolone: influence on markers of cardiovascular disease. J Clin Endocrinol Metab 1997; 82: 1752–1756

35 Rymer J, Crook D, Sidhu M, Chapman M, Stevenson JC. Effects of tibolone on serum concentrations of lipoprotein (a) in postmenopausal women. Acta Endocrinol 1993; 128: 259–262

36 Zandberg P, Peters JL, Demacker PN, Smit MJ, de Reeder EG, Meuleman DG. Tibolone prevents atherosclerotic lesion formation in cholesterol-fed, ovariectomized rabbits. Arteriosc Thromb Vasc Biol 1998; 18: 1844–1854

37 Morris EP, Denton ERE, Robinson J, MacDonald LM, Rymer JM. High resolution ultrasound assessment of the carotid artery: its relevance in postmenopausal women and the effects of tibolone on carotid artery ultrastructure. Climacteric 1999; 2: 13–20

38 Rymer J, Chapman MG, Fogelman I. Effect of tibolone on postmenopausal bone loss. Osteoporos Int 1994; 4: 314–319

39 Geusens P, Dequeker J, Gielen J, Schot LPC. Non-linear increase in vertebral density induced by a synthetic steroid (Org OD14) in women with established osteoporosis. Maturitas 1991; 13: 155–162

40 Webb P, Lopez GN, Uht RM, Kushner PJ. Tamoxifen activation of the estrogen receptor/AP-1 pathway: potential origin for the cell-specific estrogen-like effects of antiestrogens. Mol Endocrinol 1995; 9: 443–456

41 McDonnell DP, Clemm DL, Hermann T, Goldman ME, Pike JW. Analysis of estrogen receptor function in vitro reveals three distinct classes of antiestrogens. Mol Endocrinol 1995; 8: 659–668

42 Yang NN, Venugopalan M, Hardikar S, Glasebrook A. Identification of an estrogen response element activated by metabolites of 17-beta estradiol and raloxifene. Science 1996; 273: 1222–1225

43 Delmas PD, Bjarnason NH, Mitlak BH et al. Effects of raloxifene on bone mineral density, serum cholesterol concentrations, and uterine endometrium in postmenopausal women. N Engl J Med 1997; 337: 1641–1647

44 Walsh BW, Kuller LH, Wild RA et al. Effects of raloxifene on serum lipids and coagulation factors in healthy postmenopausal women. JAMA 1998; 279: 1445–1451

45 Ettinger B, Black D, Cummings S et al. Raloxifene reduces the risk of incident vertebral fractures: 24-month interim analysis. 1998;

46 Seidl MM, Stewart DE. Alternative treatments for menopausal symptoms. Can Fam Physician 1998; 44: 1299–1308

47 Bunker JP, Houghton J, Baum M. Putting the risk of breast cancer in perspective. BMJ 1998; 317: 1307–1309

48 Collaborative Group on Hormonal Factors in Breast Cancer. Breast cancer and hormone replacement therapy: collaborative reanalysis of data from 51 epidemiological studies of 52705 women with breast cancer and 108411 women without breast cancer. Lancet 1997; 350: 1047–1059

49 Daly E, Vessey MP, Hawkins MM et al. Risk of venous thromboembolism in users of hormone replacement therapy. Lancet 1996; 348: 977–980

50 Grodstein F, Stampfer MJ, Goldhaber SZ et al. Prospective study of exogenous hormones and risk of pulmonary embolism in women. Lancet 1996; 348: 983–987

51 Jick H, Derby LE, Myers MW et al. Risk of hospital admission for idiopathic venous thromboembolism among users of postmenopausal oestrogens. Lancet 1996; 348: 981–983

52 Medical Research Council's General Practice Research Framework. Randomised comparison of oestrogen versus oestrogen plus progestogen hormone replacement therapy in women with hysterectomy. BMJ 1996; 312: 473–478

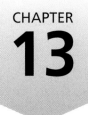

*Maria E.L. van der Burg*

# Debulking surgery in advanced ovarian cancer: the European study

Surgery plays an important role in the treatment of advanced ovarian cancer. In spite of the introduction of the more effective combination chemotherapy with platinum paclitaxel, the majority of patients with advanced stage ovarian cancer will die of recurrent disease. The worst prognosis is in patients with large residual tumour lesions after primary surgery. Already in 1975, Griffith demonstrated that patients with an optimal primary tumour debulking surgery, defined as residual lesions of less than 1.5 cm, faired significantly better.[1] Since then, many non-randomised studies showed that patients with an optimal primary tumour debulking surgery had a significant longer survival compared to patients with larger residual lesions.[2–6] The benefit of cytoreductive surgery, however, has never been demonstrated in a prospective randomised study. Despite this, primary debulking surgery is considered the cornerstone of the treatment of ovarian cancer.

## THEORETICAL BENEFITS OF CYTOREDUCTIVE SURGERY

Large tumour masses negatively influence survival. They have an adverse effect on the response to chemotherapy by the development of drug resistance.

The hypothetical rationale for increasing the survival is shown in Table 13.1. Two types of drug resistance can be distinguished: (i) temporary drug resistance, related to the size of the tumour masses; and (ii) permanent drug resistance due to the development of mutations. Temporary resistance is the result of: (i) physiological barriers; and (ii) changes in the growth rate of the tumour cells. Larger tumour masses consist of areas with poor blood supply and necrosis. These areas act as physiological barriers for cytostatic drugs.

**Dr Maria E.L. van der Burg** MD PhD, Department of Medical Oncology, University Hospital Rotterdam Dijkzigt, Dr Molewaterplein 40, 3015 GD Rotterdam, The Netherlands

**Table 13.1** Hypothetical rationale for debulking surgery

- Increase of chemosensitivity:
  - * resection areas with poor blood supply and necrosis
  - * increase of cell growth after tumour resection
  - * better diffusion of chemotherapy in small lesions
- Reduction of the development of spontaneous and drug-induced mutations
- Increase of general condition, nutrient status and quality of life

Active drugs are, therefore, unable to reach the tumour cells and an adequate diffusion of the drugs into the viable tumour cells is prevented.[7] Moreover, with the increase in the tumour volume there is a reduction in the growth rate of the tumour leading to a large number of non-proliferative resting cells. These resting cells are less sensitive to chemotherapy.[8] An important objective of tumour debulking surgery is, therefore, next to the reduction of the tumour mass, the increase in chemosensitivity of the remaining tumour cells. After resection of large tumour lesions, the growth rate of the remaining cells increases, that together with a better blood supply and better diffusion of the cytotoxic drugs into the small residual lesions, should increase the cell kill by chemotherapy.

Permanent drug resistance is caused by mutation to chemoresistant cells. These mutations arise either spontaneously or by chemotherapy. The likelihood of spontaneous and drug-induced mutation increases with growth of tumour cells.[9] Therefore, primary cytoreductive surgery may remove the already existing resistant tumour clones and reduce the development of new spontaneous mutations. Moreover, smaller tumours need less chemotherapy to be eradicated and, therefore, in smaller lesions the chance of developing chemotherapy induced-resistance is reduced.

Finally, by the reduction of bulky tumour masses, the general condition and nutritional status of the patient improves leading to a better quality of life and a better performance status. In many studies, the performance status was shown to be an independent prognostic factor for progression-free and overall survival.[3] Therefore, by tumour reduction these patients fare better.

## PRIMARY DEBULKING SURGERY

Cytoreductive surgery at primary laparotomy is accepted as beneficial for patients with advanced epithelial ovarian cancer. Most patients derive benefit from cytoreductive surgery. Patients with bulky tumours have relief of symptoms, an improvement of nutritional status, a better quality of life and a longer survival. Patients with an optimal tumour debulking surgery, in whom all residual lesions are smaller than 1 cm before the start of the chemotherapy, have a significant longer overall survival and progression-free survival than patients with larger residual lesions.[3–7] The median survival of the patients with an optimal primary debulking surgery is almost double the survival of patients with larger residual lesions. Patients in whom all macroscopic tumour is resected do have the longest survival. In the study of Michel and colleagues, the 2-year survival was 80% for patients with a radical resection of all tumour lesions, 49% for patients with lesions of 2 cm or less and 22% for the patients with lesions larger than 2 cm.[7] In the long-term, there is still a significant difference in survival. Patients with microscopic disease after primary surgery had a median survival of 6.6 years versus 1.8 years for patients with residual lesions of more than 1 cm.[3] Even in stage IV, the median survival is doubled by optimal cytoreductive surgery irrespective of the organ localisation of the metastases.[11–14] Whether the increase in survival is a result of the resection of tumour, or whether it is just the result of a selection of patients with favourable biological tumours that can be resected, has never been answered. If the tumour size of the residual lesions is the most important factor for survival, the prognosis of the patients with the same size of residual tumour lesions would be identical.

Munell and Griffiths were the first authors who demonstrated that patients in whom large tumour lesions could be resected to lesions less than 1.5 cm had the same survival as patients in whom, at diagnosis, the intra-abdominal lesions were less than 1.5 cm.[1,2,15] Recently Le and coworkers re-affirmed these findings in a retrospective study.[16] The estimated 5-year survival of 56% of 81 patients with a tumour reduction to microscopic disease was not significantly different from the 62% 5-year survival of the 24 patients with microscopic intra-abdominal disease at diagnosis. The 15% 5-year survival of 191 patients with residual lesions of more than 2 cm on the other hand was significantly lower. In another case-controlled study of 67 patients with minimal residual disease, the survival was significantly longer (4-year survival 53%) in patients in whom all the tiny peritoneal and serosal lesions were meticulously excised, compared to the survival of those (4-year survival 18%, $P = 0.003$) in whom an attempt to resect these tiny lesions was not performed.[17] In addition, Farias-Eisner and colleagues showed that the number of tiny residual lesions were an important prognostic factor for survival in patients with minimal residual disease.[18] The median survival for patients with extensive carcinomatosis was 17 months, with minimal residual nodules 31 months and without residual disease 57 months.

Hacker and coworkers, on the contrary, reported that patients with extensive intra-abdominal tumour masses did have a worse prognosis compared to patients with initial smaller intra-abdominal lesions, despite extensive tumour reduction.[19] This finding was re-affirmed in a large retrospective GOG study in small-volume stage III disease.[20] In the univariate analyses, the recurrence-free and overall survival in the 148 patients with extra-pelvic disease of 1 cm or less at diagnosis was significantly longer compared with 200 patients with large extra-pelvic disease, in spite of reduction to lesions of 1 cm or less. The median survival of the patients with primary minimal extra-pelvic disease was 64 months, versus 27.5 months for the patients with extra-pelvic disease reduction to 1 cm or less. In the multivariate analyses, the age, tumour grade and the number of rest lesions were also unfavourable prognostic factors. This indicates that, in addition to the residual tumour size, the intrinsic biological tumour factors are of importance for survival. These data, however, do not refute the beneficial effect of primary debulking surgery in advanced ovarian cancer.

The problem of all the reported retrospective non-randomised studies is the unavoidable, but serious, bias of comparing patients with different prognostic factors. The contribution of tumour reduction on survival outside prospective randomised studies is hard to define. Since a large number of studies conclude that the survival of patients with an optimal primary cytoreductive surgery is superior,[21] primary debulking surgery remains the cornerstone of treatment until the reverse is proven.

## INTERVAL DEBULKING SURGERY

Optimal primary debulking surgery in advanced ovarian cancer can, in general, be performed in around 40% of patients.[22] The prognosis of patients with suboptimal tumour debulking is poor.[4–8,22] Several retrospective studies demonstrated that, if after induction chemotherapy an optimal interval debulking surgery could be performed, the survival significantly increased.[22–24] Other studies showed no benefit from interval debulking surgery.[3,25,26] These retrospective studies compared the survival of patients with different prognostic factors. In 1993, the EORTC/GCCG showed, for the first time, that interval debulking surgery was beneficial for patients with a suboptimal primary debulking surgery.[26] In this randomised study, interval debulking surgery was an independent prognostic factor for survival as well as progression-free survival. This study was set up in 1987. The objective of the study was to answer the questions whether interval debulking surgery itself improved the progression-free and overall survival and if so which patients did benefit. Eligible were patients with advanced disease and residual lesions of more than 1 cm after primary debulking surgery.

### THE STUDY DESIGN

After informed consent, all eligible patients were registered centrally before the start of 3-weekly cyclophosphamide 750 mg/m$^2$ and cisplatin 75 mg/m$^2$. The response was evaluated after the third cycle. All patients with a response or stable disease were randomly assigned to undergo either interval debulking surgery (IDS) or no surgery after stratification for clinical response, performance status and centre. All randomised patients were to receive at least six cycles of chemotherapy. The end-points of the study were overall survival and progression-free survival (Fig. 13.1). All randomised patients were included in the analyses of progression-free survival and overall survival, which were performed strictly according to the intention to treat.

### PATIENTS

Of the 425 registered patients, 319 were randomised for interval debulking surgery (159) and no surgery (160). The patient characteristics were well balanced between the two treatment groups. The median age was 59 years, 17% of the patients had a WHO performance status 2, 21% a FIGO stage IV,

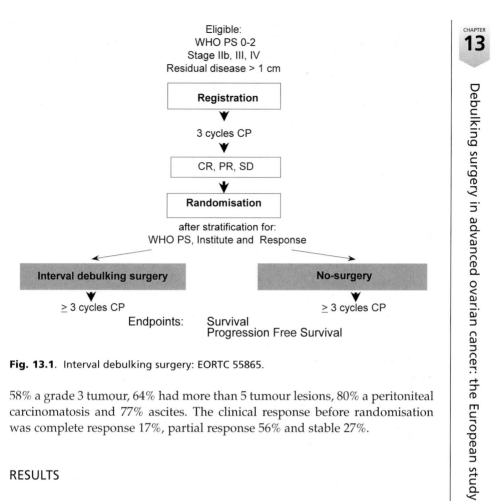

**Fig. 13.1**. Interval debulking surgery: EORTC 55865.

58% a grade 3 tumour, 64% had more than 5 tumour lesions, 80% a peritoniteal carcinomatosis and 77% ascites. The clinical response before randomisation was complete response 17%, partial response 56% and stable 27%.

## RESULTS

Of the patients assigned to interval debulking surgery, 92% underwent surgery as did 2% of the patients assigned to no surgery. The chemotherapy treatment was identical between the two groups, during the first six cycles. More patients in the no-surgery group continued chemotherapy after the sixth cycle; respectively, 56% and 41% for the no-surgery and surgery groups.

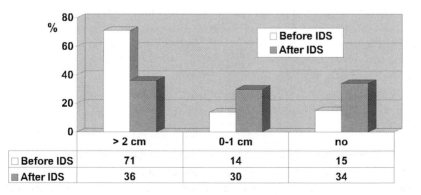

| | > 2 cm | 0-1 cm | no |
|---|---|---|---|
| Before IDS | 71 | 14 | 15 |
| After IDS | 36 | 30 | 34 |

**Fig. 13.2**. Tumour size before and after interval debulking surgery.

At interval debulking surgery, 15% of the 142 patients had no macroscopic disease, 14% had lesions of 1 cm or less and 71% had lesions of more than 1 cm. After completion of the debulking surgery, 34% had no residual tumour, 39% lesions less than 1 cm and in 36% the largest lesion was more than 1 cm (Fig. 13.2), although in almost all patients tumour reduction had been performed.

The surgical complications were minimal, and no death or severe morbidity due to interval debulking surgery was observed. The morbidity and complications were comparable in kind and severity with those observed at primary surgery and reported in the literature.[28,29]

## THE BENEFIT OF CYTOREDUCTIVE SURGERY

The effect of the cytoreductive surgery was directly translated in the response rate after six cycles of cisplatin/cyclophosphamide. The clinical complete response in the surgery group was 62% compared to 34% in the no surgery group (Fig. 13.3). In the long-term, an important benefit of the cytoreduction was observed. The survival ($P = 0.003$) and the progression-free survival ($P = 0.005$) were significantly lengthened in favour of the surgery group. The 2-year and 5-year survival was 13% and 11% higher in the surgery group (Fig. 13.4); the progression-free survival was, respectively, 9% and 7.5% higher.

The progression-free and overall survival of the patients with an optimal interval debulking surgery, resection to lesions of 1 cm or less, were not different ($P = 0.406$) from the survival of the patients who had lesions of 1 cm or less before surgery. However, a significant difference was found between patients with an optimal and non-optimal interval debulking surgery. The median progression-free survival and overall survival of the patients with an optimal tumour debulking were, respectively, 7.2 months ($P < 0.001$) and 8.5 months ($P < 0.001$) longer compared with the survival of patients with a suboptimal interval debulking surgery. It was assumed previously that patients with a suboptimal cytoreduction did not benefit from surgery. However, if we compare the progression-free and overall survival of the poor

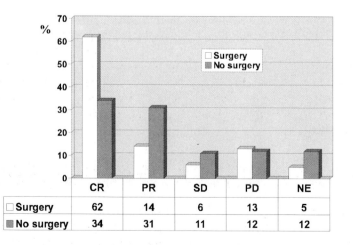

| | CR | PR | SD | PD | NE |
|---|---|---|---|---|---|
| Surgery | 62 | 14 | 6 | 13 | 5 |
| No surgery | 34 | 31 | 11 | 12 | 12 |

**Fig. 13.3.** Clinical response after 6 cycles of chemotherapy.

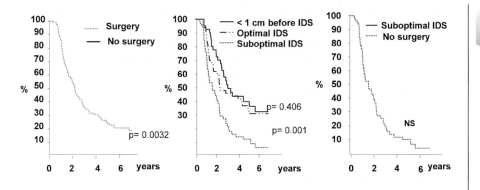

**Fig. 13.4.** Survival by interval debulking surgery: no-surgery and type of surgery.

risk patients with a suboptimal interval debulking surgery with the survival of the no-surgery patients, no difference in progression-free and overall survival was found. The median survival for the suboptimal surgery patients was 18.6 months and for the no surgery patients 19.2 months, the progression-free survival was 11.5 months each, indicating that these patients did benefit also from the interval debulking surgery (Fig. 13.4)!

In the multivariate analyses, the interval debulking surgery was an independent factor for progression-free ($P = 0.0035$) and overall survival (p= 0.0062). Moreover, after adjustment for all prognostic factors in a Cox regression model, the reduction in the risk of deaths due to surgery was 49% ($P = 0.004$). It was not possible to identify a subgroup of patients who did not benefit from interval debulking surgery. Even when patients were subdivided into a high-risk and a low-risk group, based on either individual prognostic factors or the multivariate risk, there was no difference in the relative benefit of survival between the two groups.

## CONCLUSION

In patients with residual lesions of more than 1 cm after primary cytoreductive surgery, interval debulking surgery significantly increases the progression-free and overall survival. This increase in progression-free and overall survival does outweigh the morbidity associated with interval debulking surgery. Interval debulking surgery, however, **cannot** replace the primary debulking surgery, which remains the gold standard in the treatment of ovarian cancer until proven otherwise.

## NEO-ADJUVANT CHEMOTHERAPY

Optimal debulking surgery can, in general, be performed in about 50% of patients.[21] In more experienced gynaecological oncology centres, the percentage is increased to 85%, but sometimes at the cost of an increased morbidity and sometimes mortality.[30] Several retrospective studies suggest that the

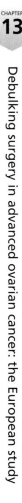

survival of patients treated with interval debulking surgery after neo-adjuvant chemotherapy is comparable to the survival of patients who underwent a primary debulking surgery, while the morbidity is lower.[24,30–32] In these studies, patient selection and comparison of patients with different prognostic factors bias these retrospective studies. The role of neo-adjuvant chemotherapy, therefore, can only be evaluated in prospective randomised studies.

The EORTC Gynecological Cancer Cooperative Group recently activated a prospective randomised study in which neo-adjuvant chemotherapy followed by interval debulking surgery is compared with primary debulking surgery followed by chemotherapy with or without interval debulking surgery. The end-points of the study are progression-free and overall survival, complication rate, morbidity, and the quality of life. Outside this study, primary debulking surgery followed by interval debulking surgery remains the standard treatment in patients with advanced bulky ovarian cancer.

---

## Key points for clinical practice

- Interval debulking surgery in advanced ovarian cancer significantly increases the survival and progression-free survival.

- Patients with tumour reduction to lesions ≤1 cm at interval debulking surgery have: (i) a significantly better survival compared to patients with larger residual lesions; and (ii) the same survival as patients with lesions ,= 1 cm before resection at interval debulking surgery.

- Patients with residual lesions > 1 cm after interval debulking surgery, patients with the worst prognosis, have the same survival as all patients in the no-surgery group. These patients with a non-optimal tumour debulking, therefore, also benefit from surgery.

- The morbidity of interval debulking surgery is the same as from primary debulking surgery.

- The reduction of the risk of death by interval debulking surgery is 49%.

- There is no difference in the reduction of death between high-risk and low-risk patients.

- Interval debulking cannot replace primary debulking surgery. Primary debulking surgery remains the cornerstone of the standard treatment of ovarian cancer until proven otherwise.

---

### Acknowledgements

The study is published on behalf of the Gynecological Cancer Cooperative Group of the EORTC and its investigators who contributed to the study: M. Van Lent, A. Kobierska, M.R. Pittelli, G. Favalli, A.J. Lacave, M. Nardi, G. Hoctin Boes, I. Teodorovic, M.A. Nooy, A. Cervantes, J.B. Vermorken, G. Bolis, L.V.A.M. Beex, C.F. De Oliveira, C. Madronal, K.J. Roozendaal, A. Poveda, M.T. Osorio, P. Zola, J.A. Wijnen, M.J. Piccart, A. Van der Gaast, and S. Pecorelli.

# References

1 Griffiths CT. Surgical resection of tumour bulk in the primary treatment of ovarian carcinoma. Natl Cancer Inst Monogr 1975; 42: 1010–1014

2 Griffiths CT, Park LM, Fuller AF. Role of cytoreductive surgical treatment in the management of advanced ovarian cancer. Cancer Treat Rep 1979; 63: 235–240

3 Neijt JP, Ten Bokkel Huinink WW, Van der Burg MEL. *et al.* Long-term survival in ovarian cancer; mature data from The Netherlands Joint Study Group for Ovarian Cancer. Eur J Cancer 1991; 27: 1367–1372

4 Omura GA, Bundy BN, Berek JS *et al.* Randomized trial of cyclophosphamide plus cisplatin with or without doxorubicin in ovarian cancer: a Gynecologic Oncology Group Study. J Clin Oncol 1989; 7: 457–465

5 Weber AM, Kennedy AW. The role of bowel resection in the primary surgical debulking of carcinoma of the ovary. J Am Coll Surg 1994; 179: 465–470

6 Bertelsen K. Tumor reduction surgery and long-term survival in advanced ovarian cancer a DACOVA study. Gynecol Oncol 1990; 38: 203–209

7 Michel G, De Laco P, Castaigne D *et al.* Extensive cytoreductive surgery in advanced ovarian cancer. Eur J Gynecol Oncol 1997; 18: 9–15

8 DeVita VT. The relationship between tumor mass and resistance to chemotherapy. Implications for surgical adjuvant treatment of cancer. Cancer 1983; 51: 1209–1220

9 Skipper H. Thoughts on cancer chemotherapy and combination modality therapy. JAMA 1974; 230: 1033–1035

10 Goldie JH, Coldman AJ. A mathematic model for relating the drug sensitivity of tumors to their spontaneous mutation rate. Cancer Treat Rep 1979; 63: 1727–1734

11 Bristow RE, Montz FJ, Lagasse LD *et al.* Survival impact of surgical cytoreduction in stage IV epithelial ovarian cancer. Gynecol Oncol 1999; 72: 278–287

12 Liu PC, Benjamin I, Morgan MA *et al.* Effect of surgical debulking on survival in stage IV ovarian cancer. Gynecol Oncol 1997; 64: 4–8

13 Curtins JP, Malik R, Venkatraman ES *et al.* Stage IV ovarian cancer: impact of surgical debulking. Gynecol Oncol 1997; 64: 9–12

14 Munkarah AR, Hallum AV, Morris M *et al.* Prognostic significance of residual disease in patients with stage IV epithelial ovarian cancer. Gynecol Oncol 1997; 64: 13–17

15 Munell EW. The changing prognosis and treatment in cancer of the ovary: a report of 235 patients with primary ovarian carcinoma 1952–1961. Am J Obstet Gynecol Oncol 1968; 100: 790–805

16 Le T, Krepart GV, Lotocti RJ *et al.* Does debulking surgery improve survival in biologically aggressive ovarian cancer? Gynecol Oncol 1998; 67: 208–214

17 Eisenkop S, Nalick R, Wang HJ *et al.* Peritoneal implant excision or ablation during cyto-reductive surgery: the impact on survival [Abstract]. Gynecol Oncol 1992; 51: 224–229

18 Farias-Eisner R, Teng F, Oliveira M *et al.* Influence of tumour grade, distribution and extent of carcinomatosis in minimal residual disease stage III epithelial ovarian cancer after optimal primary cytoreductive surgery. Gynecol Oncol 1994; 55: 108–110

19 Hacker NF, Berek JS, Lagasse LD *et al.* Primary cytoreductive surgery for epithelial ovarian cancer. Obstet Gynecol 1983; 61: 413–420

20 Hoskins WJ, Bundy BN, Thipgen T *et al.* The influence of cytoreductive surgery on recurrence-free interval and survival in small-volume stage III epithelial ovarian cancer: a Gynecologic Oncology Group Study. Gynecol Oncol 1992; 47: 159–166

21 Hoskins WJ. The influence of cytoreductive surgery on progression-free interval and survival in epithelial ovarian cancer. Baillière's Clin Obstet Gynaecol 1989; 3: 59–71

22 Neijt JP, Ten Bokkel Huinink WW, Van der Burg MEL *et al.* Randomized trial comparing combination chemotherapy regimens (HEXA-CAF vs CHAP5) in advanced ovarian carcinoma. Lancet 1984; ii: 594–600

23 Wils J, Blijham A, Naus A *et al.* Primary or delayed debulking surgery and chemo-therapy consisting of cisplatin, doxorubicin, and cyclophosphamide in stage III–IV epithelial ovarian carcinoma. J Clin Oncol 1986; 4: 1068–1073

24 Jacob JH, Gershenson DM, Morris M *et al.* Neoadjuvant chemotherapy and interval debulking surgery for advanced epithelial ovarian cancer. Gynecol Oncol 1991; 42: 146–150

25 Neijt JP, Ten Bokkel Huininck WW, Van der Burg MEL *et al.* Randomized trial comparing two combination chemotherapy regimens (CHAP5 vs CP) in advanced ovarian

carcinoma. J Clin Oncol 1987; 5: 1157–1168

26 Lawton FG, Redman CWE, Luesley DM *et al*. Neoadjuvant (cytoreductive) chemotherapy combined with intervention debulking surgery in advanced unresected epithelial ovarian cancer. Obstet Gynecol 1989; 73: 61–65

27 Van der Burg MEL, Van Lent M, Buyse M *et al*. The effect of debulking surgery after induction chemotherapy on the prognosis in advanced epithelial ovarian cancer. N Engl J Med 1995; 332: 629–634

28 Venesmaa P, Ylikorkala O. Morbidity and mortality associated with primary and repeat operations for ovarian cancer. Obstet Gynecol 1992; 79: 168–172

29 Ng LW, Rubin SC, Hoskins WJ *et al*. Aggressive chemosurgical debulking in patients with advanced ovarian cancer. Gynecol Oncol 1990; 38: 358–363

30 Vergote I, De Wever IW, Tjalma W *et al*. Neoadjuvant chemotherapy or primary debulking surgery in advanced ovarian carcinoma: a retrospective analysis of 285 patients. Gynecol Oncol 1998; 71: 413–416

31 Potter ME, Patridge EE, Hatch KD *et al*. Primary surgical therapy of ovarian cancer: how much and when. Gynecol Oncol 1991; 40: 195–200

32 Schwartz PE, Rutherford TJ, Chambers JT *et al*. Neoadjuvant chemotherapy for advanced ovarian cancer: Long-term survival. Gynecol Oncol 1999; 71: 93–99

# Index

Tibolone
  disadvantages 170–1
  for menopausal symptoms 166–7
Tocograph transducer 2
Tranexamic acid 62
Transrectal ultrasound (TRUS), in
  azoospermia 150
Tumours, drug resistance 175

## U

Ultrasound, transrectal see Transrectal
  ultrasound
Umbilical cord compression, and fetal
  hypoxaemia 14
Umbilical vein injection 60–1
Uterus
  contraction frequency determination 2–5

hyperstimulation 12
rupture 63
  and fetal hypoxaemia 14

## V

Vasal obstruction 154–5
Vascular endothelial growth factor (VEGF)
  125–126
Vascular permeability in OHSS 125
Vasography 151

## W

Weight
  gain and ovarian function 111
  loss and ovulation therapies 112–113